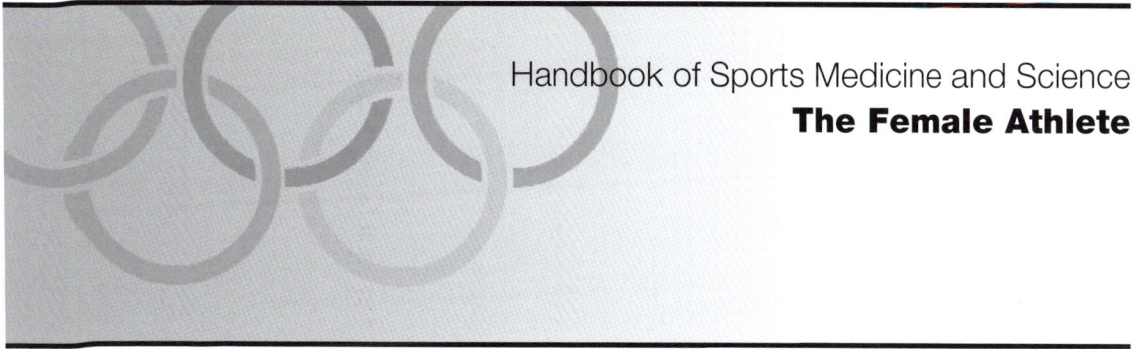

Handbook of Sports Medicine and Science
The Female Athlete

Handbook of Sports Medicine and Science

The Female Athlete

EDITED BY

Margo L. Mountjoy, MD

Assistant Clinical Professor
Director of Resident Student Affairs
IOC Medical Commission Games Group
Michael G. DeGroote School of Medicine
McMaster University, Hamilton, ON, Canada

WILEY Blackwell

For general information on our other products and services or for technical support, please contact our Customer Care Department within the United States at (800) 762-2974, outside the United States at (317) 572-3993 or fax (317) 572-4002.

Wiley also publishes its books in a variety of electronic formats. Some content that appears in print may not be available in electronic formats. For more information about Wiley products, visit our web site at www.wiley.com.

Library of Congress Cataloging-in-Publication Data:

Female athlete (Mountjoy)
   The female athlete / edited by Margo L. Mountjoy.
       p. ; cm.—(Handbook of sports medicine and science)
   Includes bibliographical references and index.
   ISBN 978-1-118-86219-3 (pbk.)
   I. Mountjoy, Margo L., editor. II. International Olympic Committee, issuing body. III. Title. IV. Series: Handbook of sports medicine and science.
   [DNLM: 1. Athletic Injuries. 2. Women's Health. 3. Athletes—psychology. 4. Sports Medicine— methods. 5. Women—psychology. QT 261]
   RD97
   617.1'027—dc23
                                                                                                    2014017661

Contents

List of Contributors

Elizabeth Arendt, MD
Professor, Department of Orthopaedic Surgery, Division of Sports Medicine University of Minnesota, Team Physician, UM Athletics, Minneapolis, MN, USA

Ruben Barakat, PhD
Professor, Faculty of Physical Activity and Sports Sciences, Technical University of Madrid, Spain

Cheri A. Blauwet, MD
Faculty, Department of Physical Medicine and Rehabilitation, Spaulding Rehabilitation Hospital/ Brigham and Women's Hospital, Harvard Medical School, Boston, MA, USA

Kari Bø, PhD
Professor, Physical Therapist, Exercise Scientist, Department of Sports Medicine, Norwegian School of Sport Sciences, Oslo, Norway

Louise M. Burke, PhD
Head of Discipline, Sports Nutrition, Australian Institute of Sport, Belconnen, ACT, Australia

Naama W. Constantini, MD
Director, Sport Medicine Center, Department of Orthopedic Surgery, The Hadassah-Hebrew University Medical Center, Jerusalem, Israel

Joan L. Duda, PhD
Professor, School of Sport, Exercise and Rehabilitation Sciences, University of Birmingham, Edgbaston, UK

Carolyn A. Emery, PhD
Associate Professor, Department of Kinesiology and Medicine, Faculty of Kinesiology, University of Calgary, Calgary, AB, Canada

Kari Fasting, PhD
Professor Emerita, Department of Social and Cultural Studies, Norwegian School of Sport Sciences, Oslo, Norway

Marci Goolsby, MD
Assistant Attending Physician, Women's Sports Medicine Center, Hospital for Special Surgery, New York, NY, USA

Suzanne S. Hecht, MD
Associate Professor, Department of Family Medicine and Community Health, Program in Sports Medicine, University of Minnesota, Program Director, UM Sports Medicine Fellowship, Team Physician, UM Athletics, Minneapolis, MN, USA

Trisha Leahy, PhD
Chief Executive, The Hong Kong Sports Institute, Sha Tin, Hong Kong

Constance M. Lebrun, MDCM
Professor, Department of Family Medicine, Faculty of Medicine and Dentistry, Glen Sather Clinic, University of Alberta, Edmonton, AB, Canada

Alejandro Lucía, MD
Professor, Universidad Europea de Madrid, Spain,
Instituto de Investigación Hospital 12 de Octubre
(i+12), Madrid, Spain

Saul Marks, MD
Division of Consultation Liaison Psychiatry,
Department of Psychiatry, University of Toronto, North
York General Hospital, Toronto, ON, Canada

Madhusmita Misra, MD
Associate Professor, Pediatrics, Endocrine and
Neuroendocrine Units, Massachusetts General Hospital
and Harvard Medical School, Boston, MA, USA

Martin Ritzén
Professor, Department of Women's and Children's
Health, Karolinska Institutet, Stockholm, Sweden

Jonatan Ruiz, PhD
Professor, PROFITH "PROmoting FITness and
Health through physical activity" research group,
Department of Physical Education and Sport, Faculty
of Sport Sciences, University of Granada, Granada,
Spain

Jorunn Sundgot-Borgen, PhD
Professor, The Sports Medicine Department,
The Norwegian School of Sport Sciences, Oslo,
Norway

Monica K. Torstveit, PhD
Associate Professor, Faculty of Health and
Sport Sciences, University of Agder, Kristiansand,
Norway

Foreword

The participation of women and girls in sport and in particular in competitive sport was slow in development throughout the ages across the entire world. Women were overlooked and often excluded from participating in competitive sport in great part because of a mistaken assumption that it was too strenuous and physically challenging.

During the past 50 years, however, there has been an explosion of interest and attention to the female athlete that has resulted in expanded opportunities for sports participation on local, regional, national, and international levels.

Women took part in the Olympic Summer Games in Paris in 1900, 4 years after the first Olympic Games of the modern era in Athens. There were 22 women out of a total of 997 athletes competing in Paris, and they took part in only 2% of the total all events. Female participation has increased steadily since then, with women taking part in 20% of the events in 1964 in Tokyo before attaining more than 46% of the events in 2012 in London, which were the first Games in which women competed in every sport on the Olympic program.

While beginning at a similarly low figure, the participation of women in the Olympic Winter Games started at 12% of the total events in 1924 at the first edition in St. Moritz, rose rapidly to 41% in 1960, and will be 50% in 2014 in Sochi.

The increased participation of female athletes in the Olympic Games and other international competition has resulted in a major increase in research activity related to sports medicine and sports science for women during the last half century. Such research has revealed the special needs of female athletes with regard to such areas as physical conditioning, nutrition, body composition, endocrinology, injury prevention and rehabilitation.

Professor Margo L. Mountjoy and a talented team of contributing authors have gathered and synthesized a large volume of information regarding the female athlete and incorporated it into this valuable Handbook. Basic and applied sciences have been combined with practical information which will be very useful, not only for medical doctors and allied health professionals, but also for team coaches and trainers, as well as athletes. We are very grateful to Professor Mountjoy for the quality of her leadership in making this publication such a highly valuable contribution to sports medicine and sports science literature.

Thomas Bach
IOC President

Preface

Female athletes around the world enjoy the health benefits of sport participation at all levels of sport ranging from the recreational level to the elite level. The XXX Olympic Games held in London 2012 saw record-setting participation for women including 4676 athletes out of 10 568 athletes (44%).

The Olympic Charter is a document that outlines the Fundamental Principles of Olympism, Rules and Bye-Law adopted by the International Olympic Committee (IOC). The Charter governs the organization, action, and operation of the Olympic Movement. The Olympic Charter mandates the promotion of women in sport:

> The IOC encourages and supports the promotion of women in sport at all levels and in all structures, with a view to implementing the principle of equality of men and women.
>
> (Rule 2, Olympic Charter in force as from July 7, 2007)

In addition to promoting the participation of women in sport, the IOC is mandated through the Olympic Charter to protect the health of the female athlete.

> The mission of the IOC is to promote Olympism throughout the world and to lead the Olympic Movement. The IOC's role is:
> ...to encourage and support measures protecting the health of athletes.
>
> (Rule 9, Olympic Charter in force as from July 7, 2007)

The Olympic Movement Medical Code which governs the actions of the IOC Medical Commission also emphasizes the importance of the protection of the health of the athlete:

> The Olympic Movement, in accomplishing its mission, should encourage all stakeholders to take measures to ensure that sport is practised without danger to the health of the athletes ... it encourages those measures necessary to protect the health of participants and to minimise the risks of physical injury and psychological harm.
>
> (Olympic Movement Medical Code 2009)

The IOC, through meeting its objective to promote Olympism and develop sport worldwide, has been active through many programs and initiatives with the goal of increasing and improving women's participation in sport at all levels over the past 20 years. The Handbook on the Female Athlete is one example of the attention of the IOC to the promotion of female participation in sport and to the protection of the health and well-being of the female athlete.

The positive health benefits of sport and physical activity for female athletes are well documented in the scientific literature. Regular physical activity through sport is shown to decrease the risk of non-communicable diseases such as diabetes, hypertension, cardiovascular disease, and some cancers. Sport also can result in psychological benefits as well as improvement in bone mineral density. There are, however, potential health risks to elite sport participation for the female athlete. This Handbook is developed to address these health risks and to provide education, as well as prevention and treatment guidelines.

The objectives of this Handbook are:

1 To increase the knowledge level of sports medicine team physicians and allied athlete health support staff of healthy female sport participation.

2 To promote safe sport participation for the women in sport by enhancing athlete entourage (coach and sport science) awareness of female athlete health issues.

3 To encourage members of the Olympic Family (International Federations and National Olympic Committees) and all sport organizations to adopt healthy female athlete practices.

The topics reviewed in this Handbook address the diverse aspects of health issues related to female sport participation. Prevention of health problems for the physically active woman includes both injuries and illnesses components. Chapters in this Handbook that focus on injury and illness prevention for the female athlete include:

• Training the female athlete
• Injury prevention
• Nutritional recommendations

To raise awareness of and to provide guidelines for the identification and management of health issues that can arise in the elite female athlete, several topic-specific chapters have been included in the Handbook. Chapters that address the potential physical health issues for the female athlete include:

• Disordered eating and eating disorders
• Bone health
• Menstrual health and contraception
• Stress incontinence
• Female athlete triad

In addition to the physical health-related topics, the Handbook also addresses the psychological health of the female athlete in the following chapters:

• Psychology of the elite female athlete
• Harassment and abuse

The final subject area that is discussed in the Handbook is the identification of unique features of special female athlete populations including:

• Gender issues and hyperandrogenism
• Exercise and pregnancy
• Paralympic athlete

Through education and implementation of healthy prevention and treatment practices outlined in the IOC Handbook on the Female Athlete, women ranging from the recreational athlete in the general population to the elite female athlete participating in the Olympic Games can look forward to enjoying the health benefits from active sport participation in the future.

I would like to acknowledge and thank the group of dedicated authors who spent countless hours writing, editing, and polishing their chapters for this Handbook. Without their expertise and devotion to the protection of the health of the female athlete, this Handbook would not have been possible.

I would also like to thank the International Olympic Committee for the recognition of the importance of the health of the female athlete. The attention of the IOC Medical Commission to this unique athlete population is important in ensuring not only healthy athletes but also improved performances at all levels of sport.

As with all large projects, the conductor is reliant on the support of the first violinist to tune the orchestra and organize the group of individual artists to perform uniformly, in time and with a consistent tone and inflection. With gratitude, I thank my first violinist—Ms. Penny Schmiedendorf of McMaster University Medical School who was instrumental in keeping this orchestra in tune.

Finally, I would like to personally thank Howard Knuttgen, the maestro of the IOC publications, for his inspiration and patient guidance in the design, development, and perfecting of this Handbook on the Female Athlete. His expertise and helpful direction is greatly appreciated.

Margo L. Mountjoy, MD
IOC Medical Commission Games Group

Chapter 1
Training the female athlete

Suzanne S. Hecht[1] and Elizabeth Arendt[2]

[1]Department of Family Medicine and Community Health, Program in Sports Medicine, Sports Medicine Fellowship, University of Minnesota Athletics, Minneapolis, MN, USA

[2]Department of Orthopaedic Surgery Division of Sports Medicine, University of Minnesota Athletics, Minneapolis, MN, USA

For the first time in Olympic history, all participating countries in the 2012 London Olympic Games had male and female athlete representation. Furthermore, greater than 40% of the London Olympic athletes were female compared to only 1.9% in the 1900 Paris Olympic Games. While great strides in female sports participation has been made, research is lacking on how to best train female athletes.

The explosion of females participating worldwide in all levels of sport continues to reach new heights. There is a need for medical providers, coaches, sport administrators, and the female athletes, themselves, to understand what constitutes optimal training for female athletes. Is training female athletes in the same manner as male athletes the best approach? The answer to this important question is unknown, but it is a fact that there are anatomic and physiologic differences (Table 1.1) between females and males and those differences may impact training. Given the limitations of our scientific knowledge in this area, it is reasonable to explore these differences and similarities and how they might impact training of male compared to female athletes in order to gain further insights on how best to train female athletes. Just as the pediatric-aged athlete is not a mini-adult athlete, female athletes are not just smaller male athletes.

Table 1.1 Physiological comparison of females and males

Physical characteristic	
Aerobic capacity (VO_2max)	M > F
Blood volume	M > F
Body fat percent	F > M
Bone mineral density	M > F
Flexibility	F > M
Muscle strength	M > F
Thermoregulation	F = M

Anatomic and physiologic considerations

Aerobic performance

Aerobic capacity in female athletes is typically 10% lower than male athletes when normalized for lean body mass. Factors contributing to a lower aerobic capacity in women are smaller hearts and thoracic cavities with smaller lung volumes, less blood volume, fewer red blood cells, and less hemoglobin. The gap in female endurance performance records compared to males is narrowing for marathons and triathlons, but may not equalize due to inherent differences in body composition and aerobic capacity.

Anaerobic performance

Females have a lower maximal anaerobic threshold than males, which may be due to differences in muscle mass and/or training differences.

Anatomic differences

Pubertal and skeletal maturation is attained at a younger age in females. On average, men are taller and have wider shoulders with narrower pelvises than women. A wider pelvis in women contributes to an increased carrying angle at the elbows and Q-angle at the knees. Women have shorter limbs and a lower center of gravity, which may offer an advantage in improved balance.

Body composition

Body fat percentage is greater in women than in men predominately due to a higher proportion of essential fat, which consists of sex-specific fat such as found in breasts, buttocks, and thighs. Storage fat is similar in both sexes.

Muscular strength

In females, total muscle mass is about 25% of body weight compared with 40% in males, and females have smaller muscle fibers. Women have a similar proportion of fast- and slow-twitch muscle fibers and make similar gains in relative muscle strength with weight training. When controlled for body weight, women have less upper body strength and similar lower body strength compared to men. Testosterone effects cause greater muscle hypertrophy in men.

Injury considerations

Non-contact ACL injury

Females have a higher risk of non-contact anterior cruciate ligament (ACL) injuries, consistent over time. Important at-risk strategies appear to be valgus collapse of the knee, with alteration in upper trunk mechanics. There is evidence that changing dynamic loading of the knee through neuromuscular proprioceptive training (i.e., avoiding at-risk positions, encouraging the knee over-the-toe position) (Figure 1.1 a and b) is of value. The recommended elements that go into ACL intervention programs include strength and power exercises, neuromuscular training, plyometrics,

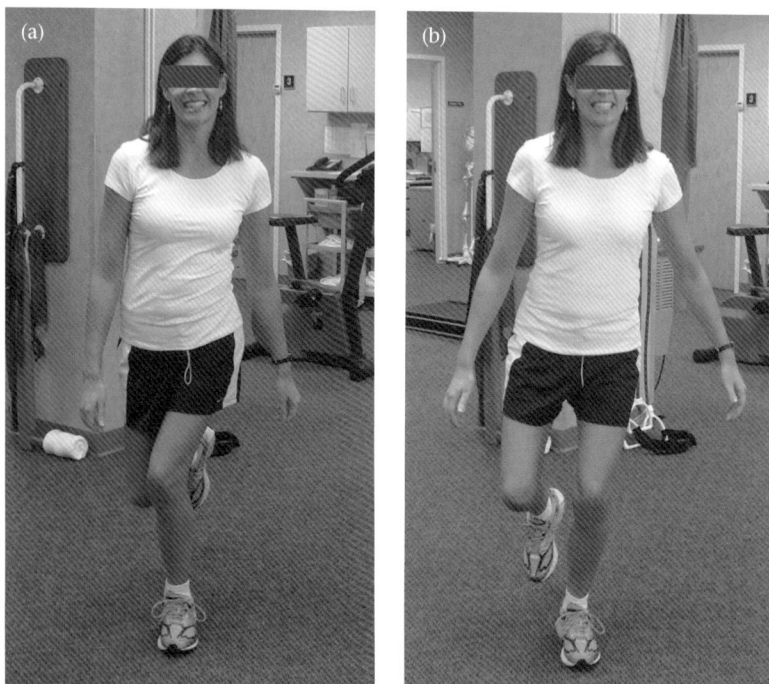

Figure 1.1 (a) Example of incorrect body movement pattern. Note the "functional" collapse of the knee when performing a partial squat, with hip substitution and pelvic drop. (b) Improved body position when performing a partial squat: hips and pelvis level, "knees over toes" position controlled throughout the knee flexion. Correct positioning mandates CORE muscle control and body position awareness.

and warm-up. The intervention formula that works best includes feedback and educational methods. Although the results are promising in existing intervention programs, the ACL injury rate and sex disparity have not yet substantially diminished through these programs. The ideal prevention program has yet to be identified.

Also somewhat disconcerting, the protective effects of ACL injury prevention programs appear to be transient. Field assessments and screening tools show promise for identifying at-risk individuals, but the best age to target the screening is not yet identified. It is unknown whether injury mechanisms and prospective risk factors are the same in the pediatric and the adult populations. More importantly, which biomechanical or neuromuscular profiles (trunk, core, hip) are most at fault in the non-contact ACL rupture remains elusive. An understanding of the causative agent is central to identifying useful screening of individuals at risk. Increasingly, there is a debate whether an ACL injury represents a gross failure of the ACL caused by a single episode or multiple episodes over time.

Females have a lower incidence of full-thickness articular lesions in ACL-injured knees. Magnetic resonance imaging (MRI) reveals a sex difference in bone edema patterns after acute ACL injury, with females more typically having posterolateral bony contusions than males. This suggests different mechanisms of injury in males versus females.

The subsequent chapter devoted to injury prevention in the female athlete and includes a detailed discussion on ACL injury prevention training programs. The assumption of a simple linear relationship between variables is unlikely to be operational in the ACL injury, as feedback loops and interrelationships are likely important. However, efforts spent on unraveling this injury mechanism is likely related to other injuries such as ankle sprains, lateral patella dislocations.

Stress fractures

Bone stress injuries result from chronic repetitive training and can range from a stress reaction to a cortical fracture. Historically, these injuries are more common in certain populations of athletes with incidence of up to 21% in track-and-field athletes and 31% in military recruits, with a female preponderance. Several evidence-based grading scales utilizing MRI have been published, which can help to grade the bone stress reaction and predict return to activities. Higher grade bone stress injuries as assessed by MRI are associated with a prolonged recovery.

General training regiments advocate activity reduction to allow pain-free activities without advocating total rest. This can follow a progression of non-weight bearing on crutches (cross-training: swimming, stationary bike, flotation running), advancing to non-pounding, weight-bearing exercises (Stairmaster™, Vancouver, Washington, Nordic Track, Logan, Utah), with gradual re-entry into sport-specific activity. Sport-specific muscle rehabilitation, strengthening, and stretching are encouraged throughout. Low-grade stress fractures can heal with continuance of activities, using pain-to-guide activities.

More recently, it has been shown that risk factors associated with the Female Athlete Triad, in particular low bone mineral density and reduced numbers of menstrual cycles, are associated with a prolonged recovery in female athletes. Athletes with trabecular bone injuries (femoral neck, pubic bone, or sacrum) more often exhibit past or present disordered eating and oligomenorrhea/amenorrhea. Those with bone stress injuries at trabecular sites had a significantly lower bone mass at the lumbar spine, femoral neck, and total hip regions.

Clinicians working with female athletes with a suspected bone stress injury need to consider the site of injury (cortical vs. cancellous) as well as the MRI grading system in management of these injuries. The medical evaluation should include a nutritional history and menstrual status. Previous training frequency and duration, and any variable offering a "change" in their previous regimen need to be evaluated and monitored during re-entry to sport.

Concussions

Epidemiological data suggest that female athletes suffer more concussions, have more severe symptoms, and take longer to recover, on average, when compared to same sport male athletes. The reason for this difference is unknown, but various theories have surfaced in an attempt to explain this difference. These theories include (1) Females have smaller head size and have less neck musculature to protect the head during impacts; (2) Female athletes are more likely to report their symptoms, although it is known that both male and female athletes under-report symptoms that are suspicious for concussion; and (3) Society is less accepting of, apt to pay more attention to, and be more concerned about head injury in female athletes compared with male athletes. On the other hand, society tends to associate sports concussions with male athletes and under-recognize its presence in female athletes.

It is currently unclear whether a strong neck protects against concussion, but consideration could be given to implementing a neck-musculature strengthening program for female athletes at increased risk of concussions. Those at increased risk include athletes that play sports with the potential for head contact with another player, ball, playing surface, or other equipment such as football (soccer), basketball, volleyball, and ice hockey. Athletes, in any sport, that have suffered one or more concussions are an at-risk group as well.

Education of the medical staff, coaches, athletes, officials, administrators, and parents about concussion signs and symptoms is beneficial in promoting early recognition and treatment. The medical staff should employ a standardized sideline assessment of any potential concussion. This would include a through medical history and physical examination, including a cognitive and a balance assessment, on any athlete suspected of having a concussion according to the Consensus Statement of the 4th International Conference on Concussion in Sport held in Zurich, Switzerland, in 2012. A recommended assessment tool for medical professionals, Sports Concussion Assessment Tool 3 (SCAT 3), and the Child SCAT for athletes younger than age 13 is available at http://bjsm.bmj.com/content/47/5/250.full. It is prudent to err on the side of caution and withhold an athlete from practice/competition if it is unclear that an athlete

has suffered a concussion, as symptoms may progress in the hours-days following a concussion. Athletes should be withheld from practices and competition until they are symptom-free and have progressed through a stepwise return to play progression without return of symptoms. Documentation of this progression is advised, including pace of progression and any player reported symptoms.

In addition to recognizing the signs and symptoms of a possible concussion, coaches can play a critical role by teaching appropriate techniques to help minimize head and neck trauma. Examples include correct football (soccer) heading technique, basketball dribbling and hockey skating with the head and eyes up rather than looking down at the ball or puck, and ball "awareness" when courtside during volleyball drills. Officials, along with coaches and administrators, can enforce and support rules that protect athletes from injury.

Medical considerations

Female athlete triad

The Female Athlete Triad describes a spectrum of three interrelated medical conditions (energy availability, menstrual health, and bone health) as defined by the American College of Sports Medicine (ACSM) in their revised 2007 Female Athlete Triad position stand. These conditions range from a healthy or optimal state (adequate energy intake, eumenorrhea, and normal bone health) at one end of the spectrum to a pathological state such as eating disorders (anorexia nervosa or bulimia nervosa), amenorrhea, and osteoporosis at the other end of the spectrum. Low energy availability (unintentional or intentional), subclinical menstrual disorders such as anovulation and luteal phase defect, and low bone mineral density lie at various points along the spectrum.

The central concept of the Triad spectrum is energy availability, which has been defined as dietary energy intake minus exercise energy expenditure normalized for fat-free mass. Simply stated, this is the number of calories remaining after the calories used for exercise have been subtracted out.

These remaining calories are used to supply fuel for everything else that a person does, including activities of daily living, growth (including bone growth), reproduction, recovery from training, cognitive function, cardiovascular function. Low energy availability can disrupt reproductive function as well as bone formation. An energy availability calculator can be found on the Female Athlete Triad Coalition web site (www.femaleathletetriad.org).

In order to avoid suffering from any of the components of the Triad, it is important for female athletes to understand their energy needs and to train and live in an environment that supports the maintenance of adequate energy availability. If an athlete is diagnosed with any one component of the Triad, it is important for healthcare professionals to assess for the other components. For a complete discussion on the triad, the reader is referred to Chapter 9.

Micronutrients for bone health

Micronutrients are critical part of an athletic nutrition plan. In addition to adequate energy availability, a variety of micronutrients are important in the diet of a female athlete. Calcium and vitamin D are of utmost importance due to the role they play in bone health. Calcium is the building block of bone and Vitamin D is critical for absorption of dietary calcium. Ninety-nine percent of the body's calcium is stored in the bone and teeth. Deficiencies of calcium and vitamin D intake are well-documented in athletes. It has been suggested, but is unknown, whether athletes need a higher level of calcium intake due to calcium losses in sweat.

The daily recommended intake of calcium for females 9–18 years old is 1300 mg/day, 19–50 years old is 1000 mg/day and 51 years old and older is 1200 mg/day. Calcium intake from dietary sources is preferred with deficits made up of calcium supplements if dietary calcium intake is inadequate. The United States' National Institutes of Health recommends a daily intake of vitamin D of 600 IU/day for females 1–70 years old and 800 IU/day for women older than 70 years.

Additional micronutrients such as vitamin K, in particular vitamin K2, along with the B vitamins and iron also play an important role in bone formation.

Chapter 6 is devoted to bone health in female athletes.

Iron deficiency anemia

The most common cause of anemia worldwide is iron deficiency. Females are at greater risk of suffering from iron deficiency anemia (IDA) than males due to iron loss from menstruation and from consuming fewer calories. Non-athletic females and female athletes have similar rates of IDA. Identifying IDA in female athletes is critical because even a mild anemia can impair performance. It is unclear whether athletes have a higher requirement for iron than the general population. Exercise has been associated with decreased serum ferritin levels (storage form of iron), depleted liver and bone marrow iron stores, and increased iron absorption and excretion.

The development of IDA in female athletes is usually due to low dietary iron intake due to inadequate caloric consumption, although an evaluation should be made to determine the underlying cause for iron deficiency as other causes of IDA exist, such as malabsorption, gastrointestinal-related blood loss, blood loss from urinary sources, or heavy menstrual cycles. Athletes should be counseled on increasing intake of foods that high in iron content and also the absorbability of iron from heme (meat) versus non-heme (plants and grains) sources. The absorption of heme iron is approximately 30% higher than from non-heme sources. Athletes following a vegetarian or vegan diet are at increased risk of IDA. Iron absorption can be improved by combining a vitamin C-containing food or beverage with the foods that are high in iron content. Avoidance of tannins (tea and coffee), carbonates, oxalates, and phosphates during meals is key, as they inhibit the absorption of non-heme iron. Iron absorption can also be inhibited by calcium, antacids, proton pump inhibitors, antihistamines, and tetracycline.

Oral iron supplements, such as ferrous sulfate or ferrous gluconate, are the mainstay of IDA treatment along with the nutritional interventions discussed above. Gastrointestinal side effects are common when taking iron supplementation;

therefore, starting slowly and gradually increasing the amount of supplemental iron is recommended. Some athletes with intolerable gastrointestinal side effects tolerate ferrous gluconate better than ferrous sulfate, which is likely due to the lower amount of elemental iron contained in ferrous gluconate. If an athlete fails to respond to oral supplementation, intravenous iron replacement can be considered assuming compliance with oral treatment and a negative investigation into a possible underlying malabsorption syndrome or other cause of continued blood loss. Intramuscular injection of iron is not recommended due to variable absorption compared to the intravenous route.

Stress urinary incontinence

Stress urinary incontinence, leakage of urine with straining, coughing, sneezing, laughing, or exercising, is a common, but typically under-reported, problem for female athletes. A study of almost 300 elite female athletes (mean age 22.8 years) from a variety of sports found that more than 40% of those surveyed had experienced leakage of urine during exercise and of those almost 10% experienced it frequently. Leakage occurred most often during jumping activities. The pregnancy and postpartum states are times of increased risk of developing stress urinary incontinence. Evidence from randomized controlled clinical trials support that pelvic floor muscle training with a physical therapist experienced in treating stress incontinence is an effective treatment method. More information on stress incontinence in female athletes can be found in Chapter 8.

Depression

It is well known that there is a higher incidence of depression in females as compared to males and this generally holds true for athletes. For athletes, both sexes are at increased risk of suffering from depression following an injury as compared to non-injured athletes although it appears that female athletes are at greater risk than their male counterparts. In light of these findings, it would be prudent for medical providers to implement screening for depression during pre-participation physicals as well as following an injury. Providing athletes access to health care providers with experience in assessing and treating depression, in addition to other mental health conditions, is recommended. Education for certified athletic trainers, physical therapists, coaching staff, and athletes in the recognition of the signs and symptoms of depression is critical to early identification of athletes at risk.

Anxiety

Females are at greater risk of being diagnosed with anxiety and tend to suffer more severe symptoms from anxiety disorders than males. Women diagnosed with anxiety disorders are more likely to be diagnosed with a comorbid mental health condition such as depression or bulimia nervosa. While data in female athletes are very limited, there is some suggestion that this increased risk of anxiety disorders holds true for female athletes. Areas of intervention include the same suggestions given above for depression but tailored to screen for and recognize signs and symptoms of anxiety disorders.

More information on psychological issues in female athletes can be found in Chapter 3.

Overtraining

As female athletes train all year round at high volumes and intensity, overtraining syndrome must be considered in the differential diagnosis for athletes that present with fatigue. Overtraining syndrome consists of the decreased or inability to perform or train at an acceptable level coupled with prolonged periods of fatigue exacerbated by exercise or activity. Numerous or recurrent infections may be a part of the clinical picture as well. While studies suggest that approximately 10% of athletes suffer from overtraining syndrome, it does not appear that female athletes are at greater risk than male athletes.

Overtraining syndrome is a diagnosis of exclusion. An evaluation of other causes of decreased performance and fatigue should be undertaken. Treatment for overtraining syndrome consists predominately of rest for weeks to months to achieve a full recovery. Periodization of training, monitoring training volumes and performance, and setting realistic goals may help prevent over-training syndrome.

Equipment considerations

Equipment and clothing choices for female athletes has expanded as female participation in sports has grown worldwide. Availability of athletic equipment appropriate for females remains a hurdle for many countries due to financial constraints or lack of financial support of women's athletics. Appropriate size and fit of female athletic equipment that addresses the specific needs of female athletes is important for injury prevention as well as maximizing performance and competition.

An example of equipment modification for injury prevention can be found in ice hockey. Male ice hockey players wear a protective cup "jockstrap" made of a hard shell to protect the male genitals from injury. As female participation in ice hockey grew, it was realized that females needed a different style of genitalia protection, and pelvic protectors (Jill strap) were designed to fit the female anatomy (Figure 1.2).

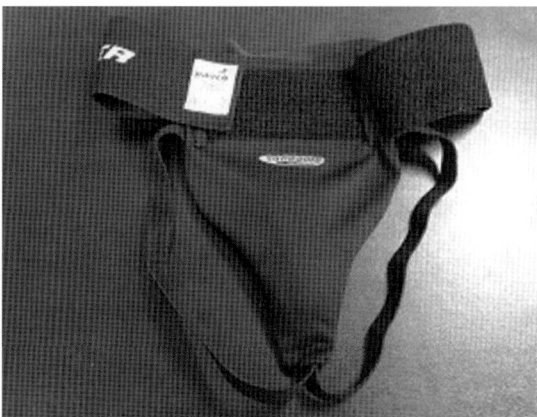

Figure 1.2 Pelvic protector (Jill strap) worn by female ice hockey players.

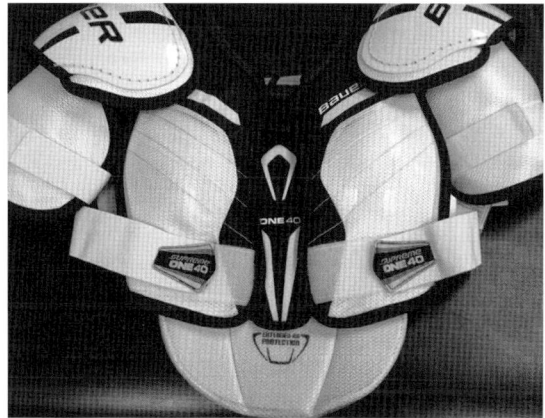

Figure 1.3 Shoulder pads and chest protector for female ice hockey players. It is designed to fit and protect the breasts.

An example of modified equipment for females that maximizes performance is found in basketball. The basketball that is used at all international women's senior-level competitions is 2.54 cm smaller in circumference than the one used by male basketball players in order to fit the smaller, on average, hand size of most female basketball players.

Breast care is an equipment issue unique to female athletes. Sports bras, available in a wide range of sizes, and specialized chest protectors (Figure 1.3) designed to accommodate breasts help to protect the breasts from injury and minimize repetitive stresses placed on the breasts.

Summary

As the science of training the female athlete continues to evolve, future research will provide more advanced insights so that we can move beyond the question: Is training female athletes in the same manner as male athletes the best approach? This will require more focused research and education on female athletes and the issues/conditions that they face in order to help them optimize their performance and health.

Recommended reading

General

Calcium recommendations. http://ods.od.nih.gov/factsheets/VitaminD-HealthProfessional/ (accessed on June 21, 2014).

Ireland ML and Nattiv A (eds). (2002) *The Female Athlete*. Elsevier Science, Philadelphia, PA.

Vitamin D recommendations. http://ods.od.nih.gov/factsheets/Calcium-HealthProfessional/

Anterior cruciate ligament

Agel J, Arendt EA, and Bershadsky B. (2005) Anterior cruciate ligament injury in National Collegiate Athletic Association basketball and soccer. *Am J Sports Med*, 33(4), 524–530.

Arendt EA and Dick R. (1995) Knee injury patterns among men and women in collegiate basketball and soccer. NCAA data and review of literature. *Am J Sports Med*, 23(6), 694–701.

Quatman CE, Quatman CC, and Hewett TE. (2009) Prediction and prevention of musculoskeletal injury: a paradigm shift in methodology. *Br J Sports Med*, 43(14), 1100–1107.

Renstrom P, Ljungqvist A, Arendt E, *et al.* (2008) Non-contact ACL injuries in female athletes: an International Olympic Committee current concepts statement. *Br J Sports Med*. 42 (6): 394–412.

Rotterud JH, Sivertsen EA, Forssblad M, *et al.* (2011) Effect of gender and sports on the risk of full-thickness articular cartilage lesions in anterior cruciate ligament-injured knees: a nationwide cohort study from Sweden and Norway of 15 783 patients. *Am J Sports Med*, 39(7), 1387–1394.

Shultz SJ, Schmits RJ, Nguyen AD, *et.al.* (2010) ACL research retreat V: an update on ACL injury risk and prevention. *J Athletic Train*, 45, 499–508.

Concussions

Center for Disease Control Concussions: http://www.cdc.gov/concussion/sports/facts.html (accessed on June 21, 2014).

Harmon KG, Drezner JA, Gammons M, *et al.* (2013) American Medical Society for Sports Medicine position statement: concussion in sport. *Br J Sports Med*, 47, 15–26.

McCrory P, Meeuwisse W, Mark A, *et al.* (2013) Consensus statement on concussion in sport: the 4th International Conference on Concussion in Sport held in Zurich, November 2012. *Br J Sports Med*, 47, 250–258.

Female athlete triad

Female Athlete Triad Coalition. www.femaleathletetriad.org/ (accessed on June 23, 2014).

Nattiv A, Loucks AB, Manore MM, *et al.* (2007) American College of Sports Medicine position stand: the female athlete triad. *Med Sci Sports Exerc*, 39(10), 1867–1918.

Sangeis P. (2006) IOC Position Stand on the Female Athlete Triad. Available online at http://www.olympic.org/Documents/Reports/EN/en_report_917.pdf (accessed on June 23, 2014).

Stress fractures

Arendt F, Agel J, Heikes C, *et al.* (2003) Stress injuries to bone in college athletes: a retrospective review of experience at a single institution. *Am J Sports Med*, 31(6), 959–968.

Nattiv A, Kennedy G, Barrack MT, *et al.* (2013) Correlation of MRI grading of bone stress injuries with clinical risk factors and return to play: a 5-year prospective study in collegiate track and field athletes. *Am J Sports Med*, 41(8), 1930–1941.

Chapter 2
Injury prevention in the female athlete

Carolyn A. Emery[1] and Constance M. Lebrun[2,3]

[1]Department of Kinesiology and Medicine, Faculty of Kinesiology, University of Calgary, Calgary, Alberta, Canada
[2]Department of Family Medicine, Faculty of Medicine and Dentistry, University of Alberta, Edmonton, Alberta, Canada
[3]Glen Sather Clinic, University of Alberta, Edmonton, Alberta, Canada

The purpose of this chapter is to provide an evidence-informed review on what is known about burden of injury, intrinsic and extrinsic risk factors, and injury prevention strategies in female athletes.

Introduction

Sport injuries in the female athlete may be predictable and potentially preventable. While one cannot eliminate all injury in female athletes, the number and severity of injuries can be reduced through various preventative strategies. With increasing involvement of female athletes at elite levels across many sports, the impact of sport injury in this population warrants attention. Reducing the risk of sport injury will have a major impact on participation in sport, performance, and long-term quality of life (QOL) through the maintenance and promotion of physical activity. There is evidence that level of physical fitness is a significant predictor of all-cause mortality, morbidity and disease-specific morbidity (e.g., cancer, cardiovascular disease, diabetes). Injuries, specifically those to the knee and ankle, are also a leading cause for the development of osteoarthritis in later life.

A four-stage approach is considered in examining injury prevention in multiple sport populations

The Female Athlete, First Edition. Edited by Margo L. Mountjoy.
© 2015 International Olympic Committee. Published 2015 by John Wiley & Sons, Inc.

and is also relevant to female athletes. First, one must understand the extent or magnitude of injury burden in female athletes and sport-specific populations prior to examining risk factors and prevention. Second, causes of injury or risk factors must be identified in the female athlete population. Third, prevention strategies need to be developed. Lastly, prevention strategies require implementation and evaluation to maximize uptake and impact in a sport-specific context.

Who is affected by injury?

Participation in sport

Females have not always enjoyed the relatively unrestricted access to sport that they currently have. In past times, the ancient Greeks actually barred women from participating at the ancient Olympics, even as spectators. No women took part in the first modern Games in 1896. Fortunately, this has changed significantly, with almost equal participation now of female and male athletes in the majority of Olympic sports. In the 2012 Summer Olympics, women's boxing made its debut, and the 2014 Sochi Winter Olympics saw the inclusion of women's ski jumping for the first time.

Over the past 40 years in particular, there has been an exponential increase in the involvement of women and girls in recreational physical activities, as well as in competitive sport at the highest levels. Women now train and compete in most sports, some in which historically only men participated. These include ice hockey, wrestling, rugby, and boxing. Participation in grassroots development in ice hockey and rugby for girls has increased significantly in the past decade (Figure 2.1). Title IX legislation in the United States (enacted in 1972, with a "mandatory compliance date" of 1978) stipulated that institutions receiving federal monies provide equal access and funding for women for extracurricular activities, opportunities for participation, scholarships, and qualified coaching. This has had a dramatic effect in the United States, with female sport participation increasing almost 10-fold over this time. The number of female professionals employed within women's athletics is at an all-time high. There have also been important and progressive advances in societal and cultural views worldwide toward the acceptance of female athletes.

Incidence of injury in female athletes (overall and sport specific)

The overall incidence of injury in female athletes varies by age, sport, level of competition, country, culture, etc., and is therefore difficult to generalize. Injury surveillance systems and tracking of injuries and their direct and indirect costs are also inconsistent between nations. It is estimated that in the United States, currently more than half of female adolescents are involved in school or club sports. Data from National Athletic Trainers' Association indicate that during a sport season more than one-third of female high school athletes experience an injury. Knee injuries represent the largest single orthopedic condition in female athletes. It is projected that among female collegiate athletes, 1 in 20 sustains a knee injury, and the risk for high school players is 1 in 50. Data from national surgical registries of Norway, Denmark, Sweden, and Germany for anterior cruciate ligament (ACL) reconstruction indicate an overall incidence of 34–81 per 100 000 citizens, with the most surgeries in the 15- to 19-year age group. This likely represents an underestimation of the true incidence, as nonoperative injuries are not captured.

The Injury Surveillance System of the National Collegiate Athletic Association has been in operation for more than 20 years. It is used to track injuries across 15 sports in a representative sample of colleges and universities (typical age of athletes of 18–23 years). A 16-year snapshot (from 1988–1989 through 2003–2004) portrayed the distribution of ACL injury, as a percentage of all injuries, and the rate per 1000 athlete-exposures (games and practices combined). Football (soccer) accounted for the greatest number of ACL injuries overall, because of

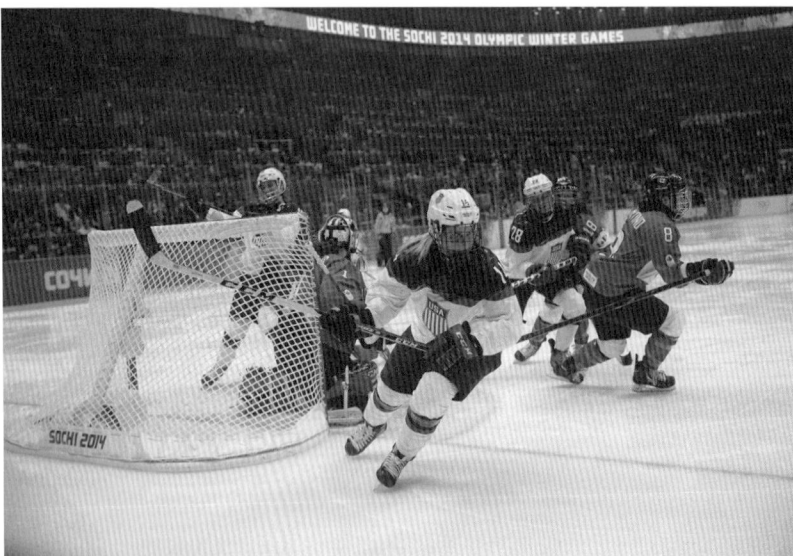

Figure 2.1 Women's ice hockey Sochi 2014 Winter Olympic Games. Final, Canada 1st; USA 2nd. ©2014/ International Olympic Committee/Chris Graythen. With permission.

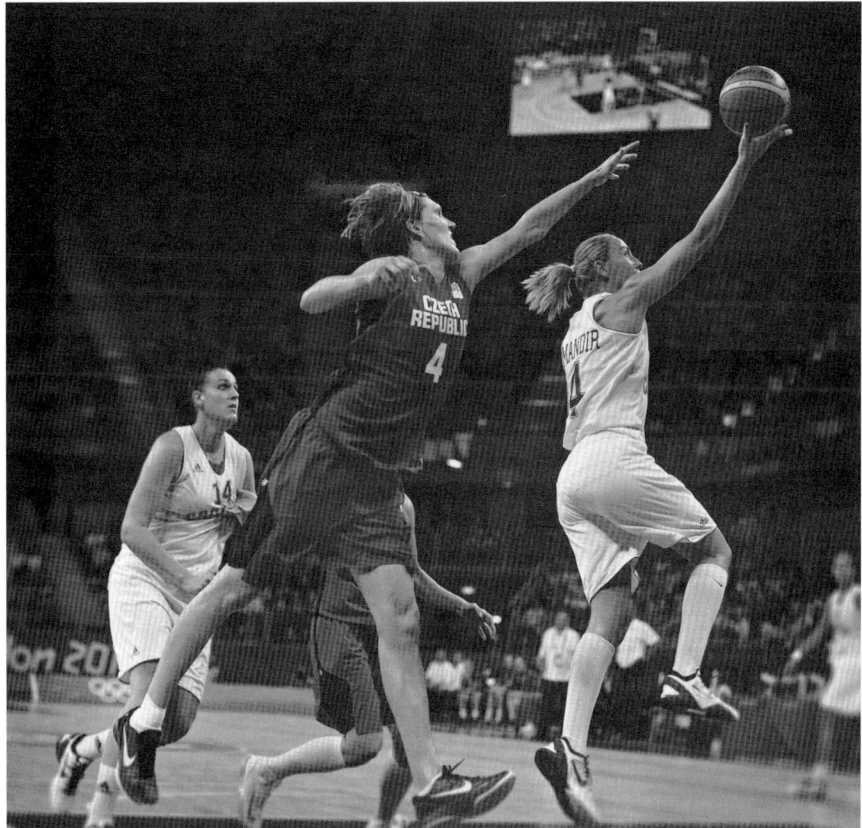

Figure 2.2 Basketball Women London 2012 Olympic Games. Qualifications, Croatia versus Czech Republic. ©2012/International Olympic Committee/ John Huet. With permission.

the largest number of participants. However, comparing the sport-specific proportion of all injuries that are ACL injuries with other injuries, female football/soccer, lacrosse, gymnastics, and basketball predominated. For the age group younger than college (14–18 years), the rate of noncontact ACL injuries in soccer was twice as high in females than in males, and in basketball, nearly four times that of males (Figure 2.2). At the professional level, the ratio of ACL injuries in male compared with female athletes approximates one; however, it is difficult to interpret whether or not this represents a true decrease. One could speculate that at least it is partly due to dropout of the previously injured players (e.g., "survival of the fittest").

In other sports, such as competitive alpine skiing, the incidence rate in females is twice that of males (Figure 2.3). Female athletes in team handball are also at extremely high risk, with the greatest incidence occurring at the most elite level of competition (Figure 2.4). Across all sports, the risk of injury is significantly greater during competition than during training.

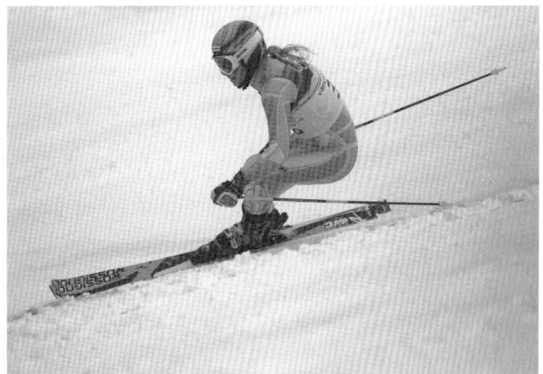

Figure 2.3 Alpine skiing, Giant slalom women Vancouver 2010 Winter Olympic Games. Ana Drev (SLO). ©2010/International Olympic Committee/Mine Kasapoglu. With permission.

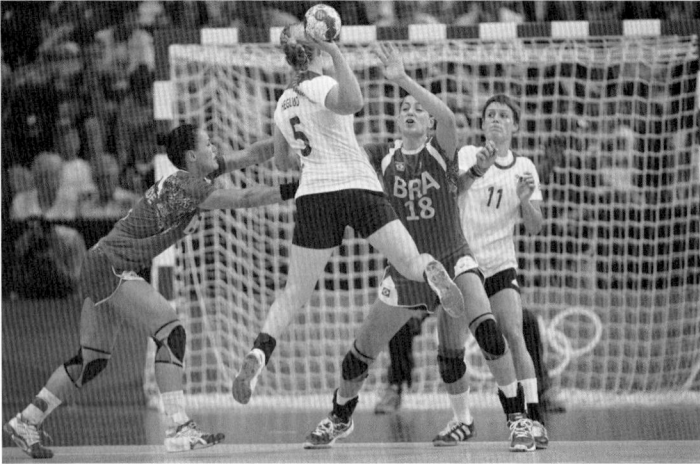

Figure 2.4 Handball Women London 2012 Olympic Games. ©2012/ International Olympic Committee/John Huet. With permission.

Where does injury occur?

Injury risk is largely sport specific, but there are some differences between males and females in specific sports. Young female athletes in gymnastics, dancing, and figure skating frequently experience spine injury including spondylolysis (Figure 2.5). Male athletes in football, ice hockey, and soccer may also experience spondylolysis. Injuries in both sexes may be either acute and traumatic, or chronic and related to overuse. Common musculoskeletal injuries in female athletes include ACL sprains, patellofemoral joint (PFJ) dysfunction and stress fractures. Previously, women were thought to have decreased upper body strength compared with their male counterparts, thus accounting for increased risk of

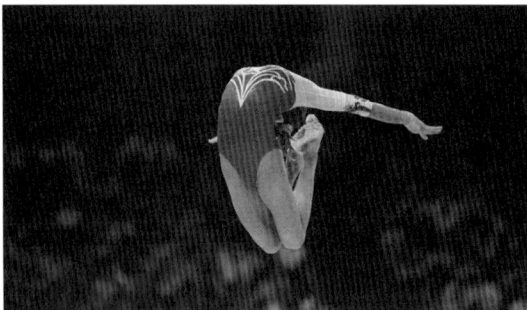

Figure 2.5 Artistic gymnastics London 2012 Olympic Games. Women team competition final. ©2012/ International Olympic Committee/John Huet. With permission.

upper extremity injury. However, earlier participation in sports by girls, as well as more adequate and sport-specific training programs has helped to moderate but not eliminate this discrepancy.

Women typically (but not always) have increased general joint laxity as compared with men. Laxity about the ankle joint and elbow is thought to lead to a greater incidence of ankle sprains and lateral epicondylitis. Interestingly, in terms of stability of the glenohumeral joint—women have increased anterior laxity, while men have increased posterior laxity. The hormone relaxin has a significant role in ligament and tendon laxity. During pregnancy, it increases ligamentous laxity to specifically facilitate changes in the sacroiliac joints and symphysis pubis, thus allowing for enlargement of the pelvic outlet during childbirth. It can also affect other ligaments, and as higher relaxin levels persist into the puerperium, women are consequently more prone to ligamentous injuries both during and immediately after pregnancy.

The majority of the literature on specific injury risks in female athletes is commonly focused on noncontact ACL injuries. Female athletes are known to have a greater propensity for lower extremity injury, in particular ACL rupture, in landing and cutting sports, such as basketball and soccer. They are reportedly at greater than threefold risk of ACL injury than male athletes in some sports. The sport-specific relative risks are 3.5 for basketball and 2.7 for soccer, both sports that are played with the same rules as their male counterparts. This is a devastating problem, leading to later life development of meniscal tears and post-traumatic osteoarthritis. In addition to decreased ability to participate in sport, the economic implications in terms of time loss from school/work, costs of operative intervention, and rehabilitation are staggering. Thus, prevention is paramount.

Predisposing causes for ACL injuries include both anatomic and physiological factors. The intercondylar notch is smaller in females, as is the ACL. Women have decreased muscle strength ratios between the quadriceps and hamstring groups, predominately utilizing the quadriceps to stabilize the knee joint, as compared with males, where hamstring activity dominates. Greater testosterone levels in men lead to larger and stronger muscles. Women are more dependent upon the strength of the ligaments, whereas males can rely more on the strength of their thighs. Possible hormonal contributing factors will be discussed subsequently.

Injuries to the PF joint are commonly attributed to different body habitus in female athletes such as wider hips and pelvis, increased femoral anteversion, and Q angle (Q angle, the angle formed by a line drawn from the anterior superior iliac spine to the center of the patella, and a line drawn through the center of the patella and the tibial tuberosity). However, scientific proof supporting this anatomic theory is limited, and a number of studies have actually documented narrower pelvic width in some females compared with males. There is evidence however to support biomechanical risk factors for PF joint injury, including altered pelvic-stabilizing abilities and landing mechanics (e.g., more erect posture, greater knee flexion excursion, greater knee flexion velocities, greater knee valgus, greater ankle contribution to energy dissipation during landing). Many of these differences are amenable to informing specific prevention programs, which can then be tailored to individual sports.

Stress fractures can account for up to 20% of all injuries treated in sports medicine clinics and lead to pain, reduced performance, lost time from training and competition and medical expense. An increased overall incidence of stress fractures has been documented in females compared with males in both athletic populations (9.7% vs. 6.5%) and military recruits (9.2% vs. 3%), with differing sites between the sexes. These are seen in the tibia in both men and women and can also occur in nonweight-bearing

extremities and the ribs, depending upon sport-specific loads. Women tend to have more stress fractures in the femoral neck, tarsal navicular, metatarsal, and pelvic bones (Figure 2.6).

The alterations in reproductive hormones that occur throughout a female athlete's life cycle (e.g., menarche, menstrual cycles, pregnancy and parturition, menopause) have been postulated to have a variety of effects on substrate metabolism, cardiorespiratory function, and thermoregulation, as well as on psychological factors and musculoskeletal injury rates. The latter two may sometimes be related. However, actions of the individual endogenous sex steroids (estradiol and progesterone) can be antagonistic, synergistic or additive, making research in this area extremely complex and difficult to carry out. The addition of exogenous hormones in oral contraceptives (OCs) and hormone replacement therapy further complicates accurate scientific studies. Of note, however, is the fact that world records have been set, and Olympic medals won at any phase of the menstrual cycle.

Nevertheless, this continues to be a "fertile" field for scientific investigation. For example, subsequent to the discovery of receptors for both estrogen and progesterone (as well as for testosterone and relaxin) in the ACL ligaments themselves, a number of researchers have postulated increased

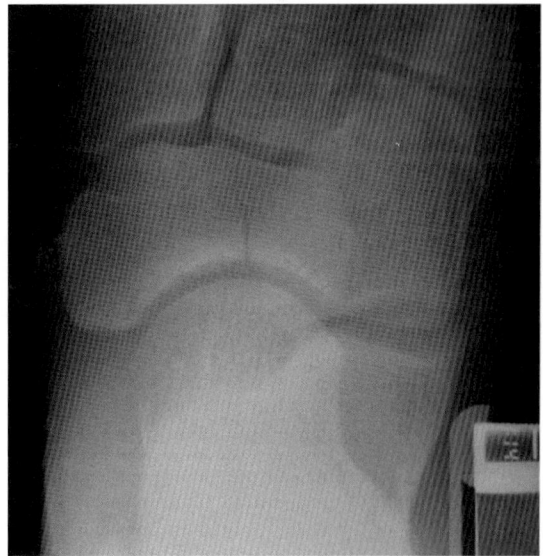

Figure 2.6 Navicular stress fracture.

risk of ACL rupture in female athletes during the pre-ovulatory phase, when both hormones are high. Knee valgus, a known ACL injury risk factor, is also thought to be subject to hormonal changes during the menstrual cycle. Research is ongoing and continues to suggest a greater risk around this point in the menstrual cycle, but to date, there is no definitive proof that altering the menstrual cycle by the administration of exogenous hormones, such as OCs, is beneficial in terms of injury reduction.

As well, elite female athletes who train intensely are at risk of developing functional hypothalamic amenorrhea (FHA), due primarily to inadequate energy intake. This can be either deliberate (as in disordered eating and the frank eating disorders of anorexia nervosa and bulimia nervosa) or inadvertent, with insufficient replacement of energy for exercising needs. The subsequent menstrual dysfunction and chronic estrogen deficient state, in combination with the low intake of calories and micronutrients such as calcium can lead to loss of bone mineral density (BMD). Together, these entities are termed the Female Athlete Triad, and if one of them is diagnosed, current medical practice is to actively search out presence of the others. More commonly, only one or two of these disorders coexist in any individual. Recently, endothelial dysfunction (linked to an increased risk of cardiovascular disease) has also been found to be part of the adverse health outcome in females with the triad disorders, and the term *female athlete tetrad* has therefore been suggested by some researchers. The underpinning cause, however, remains low energy availability (LEA).

The BMD changes may be simply low BMD for age or may progress further to osteopenia or frank osteoporosis, with an increased risk for fractures, including stress fractures, as discussed above. Most worrisome is the young adolescent athlete, who should be building up peak BMD during the critical years of rapid growth. There is some evidence that weight-bearing exercise is osteogenic and osteoprotective, particularly if it is repetitive, and in odd or different directions. Although this may to some extent mitigate the effects of low estrogen and caloric deficit, it is not completely protective. There is an ongoing need to educate athletes, coaches, and physicians about the triad disorders, in particular, about the significance of maintaining normal menstrual function

and adequate energy replacement, both for health and for optimal performance.

Finally, the differences in reproductive hormones between females and males may lead to disparities with respect to concussive injuries. Female athletes appear to have a greater risk of concussion, with slower recovery afterward. Girls playing high school soccer suffer concussions 68% more often than boys playing the same sport; similarly, in high school basketball, rates were almost three times higher. Based on symptom reporting, girls are more likely to report concussion. Girls also took much longer than boys for concussion symptoms to resolve and to return to play. The same patterns have been seen in collegiate soccer and basketball. Among collegiate ice hockey players, women sustain higher levels of concussions than men. They may be more prone to injury because their heads are smaller (one study of collegiate soccer players found that females had 26% less total mass in their head and neck than males) and/or because their neck muscles are less developed than boys and not as good as boys at absorbing shock of impact.

There are also differences in the number and type of postconcussion symptoms reported by female athletes, as well as in the existence of other confounders such as previous headaches, including migraines. Equally though, some of the symptoms may either be regarded as "normal," or wrongly attributed to other conditions, such as stress or depression. They may not warrant as much attention during sideline evaluations as the symptoms of male athletes with the same injury.

How does injury occur? (Mechanisms)

The most detailed characterization of injury mechanisms comes from studies of ACL injuries. As opposed to a contact or direct blow injuries (which account for less than 20% of ACL injuries), noncontact ACL injuries in female athletes appear to have two specific patterns: (i) deceleration with a planted foot, internally rotated and valgus knee, and (ii) anterior tibial shear stress from quadriceps contraction near full knee extension. Video analyses, with subsequent mapping of the kinematics, give the most accurate portrayal of injury mechanism. Recent work has been done to better standardize model-based image matching, using one or more camera views. In general, these studies show an increased knee valgus, with a straighter stiffer leg at landing at the time of injury. A "position of no return" has also been described, where the body is forward-flexed, the hip abducted, the knee internally/externally rotated with valgus, and the foot pronated. A safer landing position is with a more flexed hip and knee, and normal lumbar lordosis. This allows for improved postural awareness and a more coordinated landing. As mentioned, there are significant sex differences in patterns of neuromuscular activation, and females are more susceptible to the effects of fatigue on both muscular balance and landing mechanics. Better understanding of injury mechanisms will lead to improved knowledge about design and implementation of preventative strategies.

What is the impact of injury?

One can attempt to document the public health burden of injury in female sport according to time loss, clinical outcomes, and/or economic burden). However, these will vary by sex, socioeconomic status, country, and nationality, as well as by the specific injury, and its impact on the individual. Furthermore, the nature of data collection and reporting can give very different pictures. For example, earlier studies documented that 175 000–200 000 ACL reconstruction procedures have been conducted annually in the United States, with an estimated cost of between $115 000 and $17 000 per injury. Another interpretation, in a very recently published study, looked at the average lifetime societal benefit of ACL reconstruction surgery based on information from several large US orthopedic databases, and estimation and extrapolation of associated costs for surgical reconstruction versus structured rehabilitation. The indirect costs (as defined by lost wages, productivity, and disability) in a patient with a symptomatic unstable knee after an ACL injury are substantial. However, the longer term societal costs associated with degenerative osteoarthritis and/or knee arthroplasties are also significant. Patients with no meniscal tear have a 0–13% risk of developing knee osteoarthritis at ten years after injury, whereas those with a meniscal tear have a 21–48% risk. Factoring in the costs of ACL reconstruction surgery (including rehabilita-

tion afterward) versus conservative management (i.e., rehabilitation), it was put forth that in the short-to-intermediate term (up to 6 years), ACL reconstruction was more effective and had an overall cost reduction of $4503 per patient. In the long-term, mean incremental cost savings were postulated to be $50 000 per patient, with an incremental gain in QOL compared with rehabilitation. The majority of the societal savings came from the patient's ability to return to a more functional and pain-free lifestyle and by minimizing any further damage to the knee that would lead to the development knee osteoarthritis in the future. In fact, the authors estimate lifetime societal savings in the United States of about $10.1 billion for the ACL surgeries annually.

Although many female athletes are able to return to sport after appropriate surgical management of injuries and/or rehabilitation, it is difficult to identify the number who cannot, or who return, but at a lower level of function. There is an extremely high risk of secondary injuries after the initial injury, and another potential problem for young athletes is the risk of growth disturbances when reconstruction is performed before puberty. As mentioned, long-term studies have shown that approximately 50% of patients will have radiographic osteoarthritis 15 years after an ACL injury, independent

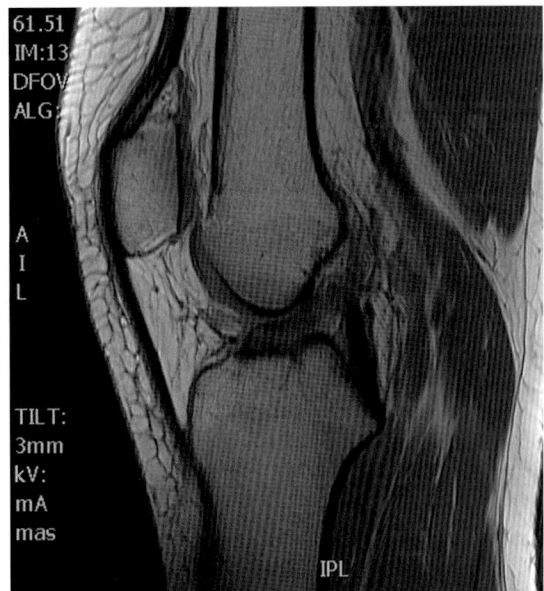

Figure 2.7 MRI of knee with ACL tear.

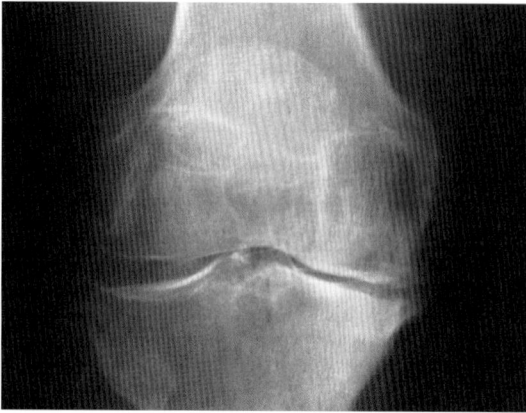

Figure 2.8 X-ray of significant medial OA of the knee.

of treatment (Figures 2.7 and 2.8). There is no evidence in the literature that rehabilitation after ACL reconstruction should be different for both men and women. What is known, however, is that prevention of such injuries remains economically more beneficial than any kind of treatment.

What are the risk factors for injury in female athletes?

Risk factors in sport are any factors that increase the potential for injury. They may be either extrinsic (i.e., rules of the sport, playing surface, equipment used) or intrinsic (i.e., age, strength, balance) to the athlete. Modifiable risk factors are those that can be altered by injury prevention strategies to reduce injury risk. Nonmodifiable risk factors, which cannot be altered, may affect the association between modifiable risk factors and injury (e.g., sex may differentially impact the relationship between baseline symptoms including headache, neck pain, dizziness, and concussion risk). Identification of these various factors will assist in defining high-risk populations. Potential risk factors for injury in child and adolescent sport are listed in Table 2.1. Similar issues exist in adult female athletes, with increasing age and history of previous injury becoming more prominent as causes of and contributors to injury.

Table 2.1 Potential risk factors for injury in child and adolescent sport

Extrinsic risk factors	Intrinsic risk factors
Nonmodifiable • Sport played (contact/no contact) • Level of play (recreational/elite) • Position played • Weather • Time of season/time of day	Nonmodifiable • Previous injury • Age • Sex
Potentially modifiable • Rules • Playing time • Playing surface (type/condition) • Equipment (protective/footwear)	Potentially modifiable • Fitness level • Preparticipation in sport-specific training • Flexibility • Strength • Joint stability • Biomechanics • Balance/proprioception • Symptoms (e.g., headache, dizziness, neck pain) • Psychological/social factors

Much of the literature addressing sport injury in female athletes is sport specific and based on descriptive data that portray primarily the extent of the injury problem. There is a growing body of literature demonstrating that risk factors are identifiable for sport injuries in the elite athlete population; however, fewer studies focus on the female athlete. The evidence for injury prevention strategies reducing the risk of injury in female athletes is based primarily on cohort studies for specific injuries in specific sports.

Nonmodifiable risk factors for injury in the female athlete

In identifying nonmodifiable risk factors for injury in elite athletes, there is evidence that males overall may be at a greater risk for injury, with the exception of soccer and basketball where females are at a greater risk. Male athletes may have a larger body mass and resultant greater forces and experience greater contact in some sports compared with females participating in the same sports (e.g., ice hockey). The higher risk of injury in some sports such as soccer and basketball may also be of a physiological nature. For example, women have greater than threefold increased risk of sustaining an ACL injury than men playing the same sports, with the same rules. As noted above, the reasons for this may be biomechanical and/or physiological in nature.

Re-injury rates are high in elite female competitive athletes. The risk of re-injury in most sports is greater than the risk of first-time injury. Previous injury increases the risk of subsequent injury in sport. This finding may be related to persistent symptoms, underlying physiological deficiencies resulting from the initial injury (i.e., ligamentous laxity, muscle strength, endurance, proprioception), inadequate rehabilitation, or perhaps a biological predisposition. There are some reports suggesting specific biomarkers as predictive of specific injury types (e.g., concussion).

Sport-specific rates of injury vary considerably with the highest rates of injury reported in wrestling, ice hockey, soccer, European handball, basketball, athletics, and gymnastics. In female Paralympic sport, the highest rates of injury are reported in goalball, athletics, and wheelchair basketball. It is not surprising that ice hockey, soccer, handball, and basketball are consistently among the top-rated sports for injury in female athletes. These sports involve a high rate of player-to-player contact, speed, pivoting, and jumping/landing (with ice hockey being the exception), which are often involved in the mechanism of injury. It is also somewhat predictable that wrestling and gymnastics are also consistently among the top-rated sports for injury in female athletes, with athlete-to-athlete contact in wrestling, high levels of jumping, landing and sprinting in gymnastics, and high training loads and pivoting activities in both sports.

Risk of injury increases with greater exposure to competition and training (hours of participation), competition (compared to training), tournament play (compared to regular season play), and increased level of competition. Athletes may be exposed to greater stress, greater intensity, and higher speeds and contact in competition and tournaments compared to training and regular season competition, thus increasing the risk of sustaining an injury.

There is conflicting evidence regarding anthropometric measurement and risk of injury which appears to be injury and sport specific. In gymnastics and soccer, athletes who are taller or heavier may be at an increased risk compared with those who are shorter or lighter. It may be that taller and heavier athletes are more susceptible to injury due to greater forces being absorbed through soft tissue and joints. In ice hockey, smaller players may be more susceptible to injury. Although skeletal maturity may not in itself be a risk factor that can be altered, in the context of sport, it may be a modifiable risk factor in some sports such as gymnastics, where adjusted training loads may be considered in skeletally immature female athletes.

Potentially modifiable risk factors for injury in female athletes

Biomechanical alignment may be a risk factor for injury in running and jumping sports. Side-to-side asymmetries in kinetics and kinematics and hip and knee alignment on a vertical drop jump test may be associated with greater knee injury risk in female running and jumping athletes. There is some evidence of an association between poor flexibility and injury in figure skating and gymnastics, where there is a high degree of flexibility required for execution of many maneuvers. Decreased flexibility is not a risk factor generally for injury in sport. On the contrary, increased shoulder ligament laxity has been shown to be associated with an increased risk of shoulder injury in some sports such as wrestling and swimming.

Fatigue may play a role in some sports where there is an increased risk of injury reported in the period of time close to the end of competition (e.g., soccer and athletics). Decreased levels of endurance fitness may also be associated with injury risk (e.g., muscle strain injury). Injury risk may be greater with decreased levels of endurance and/or strength associated with limited sport-specific preseason training. Some female athlete populations (i.e., low-skill division adolescent female soccer players) may benefit more from training programs than others (i.e., high-skill division adolescent female soccer players). Balance training, in conjunction with other neuromuscular training components, has been shown to reduce the risk of lower extremity injuries in soccer, European handball, and basketball. The impact of decreased balance as a risk factor for injury however remains unclear.

Psychosocial risk factors may also be potentially modifiable. Lower socioeconomic status may be predictive of injury. Studies consistently report a significant association between injury in sport and life stress.

Injury prevention in female athletes

The injury prevention strategies in female athletes that have had the most attention in the literature are multifaceted neuromuscular training programs to prevent lower extremity injuries. These specifically target risk factors such as limitations in proprioception/balance, jumping/landing technique, strength, endurance, and flexibility. Overall, studies suggest a protective effect of such programs on primarily acute onset injuries (e.g., ankle sprain, ACL ligament sprain) in sports with a significant amount of running/jumping/pivoting activities (e.g., soccer, handball, basketball). Further, there is evidence to suggest an impact of such injury prevention programs on improvement of skill performance (e.g., functional balance) in soccer. In soccer, there is some evidence that the protective effect of such a program is more effective in lower skilled players compared with more elite players. There is also evidence to suggest that ongoing adherence and maintenance of such neuromuscular training programs is limited, despite the association between levels of adherence and magnitude of effectiveness in reducing the risk of injury. Current research is focusing on programs that will influence behavioral change to maximize adherence and maintenance of such injury prevention programs.

There is evidence to support decreased muscle strength (e.g., hamstring injury in soccer), decreased sport-specific training (e.g., groin injury in ice hockey), previous injury, and decreased endurance as significant risk factors for muscle strain injury in sport. Sport-specific and eccentric strength training components may be essential components of a neuromuscular training prevention program in reducing muscle strain injuries specifically.

Previous injury is consistently reported as a primary risk factor for injury in female athletes in all sports. In addition, there is increased evidence to support identification of sport- and sex-specific risk factors. As such, it is imperative to consider preseason musculoskeletal screening and appropriate individually targeted rehabilitation as an important approach to injury prevention in both female and male athletes.

Protective equipment in many sports (e.g., full-face masks and mouth guards in ice hockey, shin pads in soccer, helmets in cycling, skiing, and snowboarding) has been shown to exert a protective effect. While there is a paucity of research evaluating the appropriate fitting and protective effect of such gear specifically in female athletes, there is evidence to support the effectiveness of equipment such as helmets more broadly, as well as the development of sport rules and regulations that align together. Ankle bracing or taping in combination with neuromuscular training following ankle sprain injury may play an important role in reducing the risk of re-injury following an ankle sprain. In addition, attention to rules of play and enforcement (e.g., body checking in ice hockey, illegal play in soccer and basketball, head contact) is key in preventing injuries across multiple female sports.

Conclusions and future research in injury prevention in pediatric sport

Female participation rates and injury rates in sport are high. Injury in sport will affect future involvement in physical activity and the ultimate health of these athletes. The long-term impact of joint injury (e.g., meniscus and ACL injury) in the development of early degenerative osteoarthritis of the knee is clear. Future research should focus on primary and secondary prevention of injury, but also on tertiary prevention to prevent the negative health effects of inactivity and early osteoarthritis.

The strength of the evidence for potentially modifiable intrinsic risk factors for injury (e.g., balance, strength, endurance) in female athletes has led to the development and evaluation of effective multifaceted neuromuscular training strategies to reduce the risk of injuries in female athletes. Further research examining psychosocial factors, overtraining, sleep patterns, nutrition and extrinsic risk factors (e.g., playing surface, rules, equipment) is warranted.

Future studies evaluating sport-specific injury prevention strategies must consider a multifaceted approach to prevention. It is crucial to integrate basic science, clinical, and epidemiological research to maximize the understanding of mechanisms of injury, risk factors for injury, optimal prevention strategies, and long-term effects of injury. Comprehensive and longitudinal follow-up studies are critical to the understanding of lasting effects of injury in female athletes. Finally, the emerging field of implementation science in sports injury prevention has much to offer in this field.

Recommended reading

Acosta RV and Carpenter LJ. (2012) Women in intercollegiate sport: a longitudinal, national study thirty-five year update 1977–2012. Unpublished manuscript. Available at http://acostacarpenter.org/AcostaCarpenter2012.pdf (accessed on May 13, 2014).

Chen Y-T, Tenforde AS, and Fredericson M. (2013) Update on stress fractures in female athletes: epidemiology, treatment and prevention. *Curr Rev Musculoskelet Med*, 6, 173–181.

Collard DCM, Verhagen EALM, van Mechelen W, Heymans MW, and Chinapaw MJM. (2011) Economic burden of physical activity-related injuries in Dutch children aged 10–12. *Br J Sports Med*, 45, 1058–1063.

Daneshvar DH, Nowinski CJ, McKee A, and Cantu RC. (2011) The epidemiology of sport-related concussion. *Clin Sport Med*, 30(1), 1–17.

De Souza MJ, Nattiv A, Joy E, *et al.* (2014) 2014 Female Athlete Triad Coalition Consensus Statement on Treatment and Return to Play of the Female Athlete Triad: 1st International Conference held in San Francisco, California, May 2012 and 2nd International Conference held in Indianapolis, Indiana May 2013. *Br J Sports Med*, 48(4), 289–309.

Doherty C, Delahunt E, Caulfield B, Hertel J, Ryan J, and Bleakley C. (2014) The incidence and prevalence of ankle sprain injury: a systematic review and meta-analysis of prospective epidemiological studies. *Sports Med*, 44(1), 123–140.

Donaldson A and Finch CF. (2013) Applying implementation science to sports injury prevention. *Br J Sport Med*, 47(8), 473–475.

Gagnier JJ, Morgenstern H, and Chess L. (2013) Interventions designed to prevent anterior cruciate ligament injuries in adolescents and adults: a systematic review and meta-analysis. *Am J Sports Med*, 41(8), 1952–1962.

Hootman JM, Dick R, and Agel J. (2007) Epidemiology of collegiate injuries for 15 sports: summary and recommendations for injury prevention initiatives. *J Athl Train*, 42, 311–319.

Ireland ML. (2002) The female ACL: why is it more prone to injury? *Orthop Clin North Am*, 33, 637–651.

Mather RC III, Koenig L, Kocher MS, *et al.* (2013) Societal and economic impact of anterior cruciate ligament tears. *J Bone Joint Surg*, 95A(19), 1751–1759.

Meeuwisse WH, Tyreman H, Hagel B, and Emery C. (2007) A dynamic model of etiology in sport injury: the recursive nature of risk and causation. *Clin J Sport Med*, 17(3), 215–219.

Mountjoy M, Sundgot-Borgen J, Burke L, *et al.* (2014) The IOC consensus statement: beyond the Female Athlete Triad – Relative Energy Deficiency in Sport (RED-S). *Br J Sports Med*, 48(7), 491–497.

Renstrom P, Ljungqvist A, Arendt E, *et al.* (2008) Non-contact ACL injuries in female athletes: an International Olympic Committee current concepts statement. *Br J Sport Med*, 42(6), 394–412.

Smith HC, Vacek P, Johnson, RJ *et al.* (2012) Risk factors for anterior cruciate ligament injury: a review of the literature—Part 2: hormonal, genetic, cognitive function, previous injury, and extrinsic risk factors. *Sports Health*, 4(2), 155–161.

Wentz L, Liu PW, Haymes E, and Ilich JZ. (2011) Females have a greater incidence of stress fractures in both military and athletic populations: a systematic review. *Mil Med*, 176, 420–430.

Yank J, Tibbetts AS, Covassin T, *et al.* (2012) Epidemiology of overuse and acute injuries among competitive collegiate athletes. *J Athl Train*, 47(2),198–204.

Chapter 3
Psychology of the female athlete

Joan L. Duda[1] and Saul Marks[2]

[1]School of Sport, Exercise and Rehabilitation Sciences, University of Birmingham, Edgbaston, UK
[2]Division of Consultation Liaison Psychiatry, Department of Psychiatry, University of Toronto, Toronto, Ontario, Canada

Introduction

The field of sport psychology is concerned with the psychological factors and social psychological processes impacting sport performance and participation of athletes and athletic teams at all competitive levels. Sport psychology, as a scientific discipline and area of applied practice, has grown significantly over the past 50 years. The number of and membership comprising professional organizations in sport psychology around the world (e.g., the International Society of Sport Psychology; the Association of Applied Sport Psychology), and scientific publication outlets for research in this area (e.g., the *Journal of Sport and Exercise Psychology, Psychology of Sport and Exercise*), have increased. The relevance of the field to maximizing training and competitive performances is now more widely recognized and accepted. Athletes and their coaches are more aware that the regular practicing of psychological techniques and the systematic development of psychological skills should go "hand in hand" with physical training and physical preparation for competition. It is recommended that athletes formulate and consistently rehearse (in training) and apply (in competition) preperformance and postperformance routines that are comprised of physical (e.g., when at the free throw line, several bounces of the basketball and

then a deep breath before shooting) and psychological (e.g., "seeing" and "feeling" where the shot will go and committing to that goal) components.

Research in sport psychology also speaks to the importance of the coach-created environment to the quality of athletes' sport engagement and the likelihood of their maintaining participation. Theory- and evidence-based training programs now exist, which 'set the stage' for more positive and adaptive (and less negative and maladaptive) exchanges between athletes and their coaches and other significant others in their lives, such as parents.

Sports psychiatry has often been a misunderstood and under-serviced area of medicine in the world of sport. Sports psychiatry made its defining entry into the scientific literature in May 1992, in the *American Journal of Psychiatry*, in a paper titled "An Overview of Sport Psychiatry" by Dr. Daniel Begel. As a medical specialty, psychiatry has been recognized since the middle of the nineteenth century; however, the interface between psychiatry and the world of sport has often been misunderstood. Dr. Begel defined sport psychiatry as the implementation of psychiatric knowledge and treatment methods to the world of sport. Elite athletes are subject to massive somatic, social, and mental stress. Although the public has great interest for athletic achievements, the emotional strains brought on by such "heroic moments" until the last two decades have not been considered in the scientific literature. Over time, there have been more and more papers in research journals and presentations at international scientific conferences on the subject. The field, however, has suffered from a lack of controlled studies (and data) on incidence, phenomenology, and treatment of psychiatric disorders in athletes.

In this chapter, we summarize some of the latest findings stemming from the fields of sport psychology and sport psychiatry, which relate to female athletes' functioning within the sport setting, their psychological and physical health, and overall well-being. We conclude by calling for integrative research approaches that can inform evidence-based and interdisciplinary practice in optimizing the psychology of female athletes and addressing the mental health issues faced by them.

The importance of mental skills training

Sport psychology emphasizes the importance of helping athletes learn and become proficient at psychological techniques (such as goal setting, positive self-talk, imagery, the use of focus cues, relaxation, and activation techniques) that can provide them with the skills to more effectively regulate cognitions, emotions, and behaviors during training and competitive events. This is often referred to as "mental skills training" or MST. Although more controlled trials are needed, research has revealed that elite athletes benefit from MST in terms of their performance, confidence levels, concentration capabilities, and attentional focus and/or observed decreases in debilitating anxiety. The goals of MST, however, are assumed to be much broader than performance enhancement per se. The literature indicates that systematic training that results in athletes possessing strong and robust mental skills also can lead to greater health and well-being. Most of the research to date has centered on adult-age athletes, but studies have also demonstrated that younger athletes, such as those climbing the ladder to elite levels, witness positive effects from MST. Indeed, it has been suggested that the ideal time for athletes to be introduced and gain fluency in mental skills is when they are young. In this way, young competitors are more likely to have the "mindset" to exploit their skill progression. They also would be prone to demonstrate resiliency to handle the setbacks that are inevitable as

one becomes more "serious" about sport and strives to be competing with better and better opponents.

MST and implications for athlete motivation

The literature suggests a synergy between the enhanced self-regulation capabilities, which can be developed in athletes via MST and more autonomous reasons for sport engagement. More specifically, when an athlete is more self-regulated, this athlete is more likely to be self-determined. Autonomous or more self-determined reasons include participating in sport out of personal choice and because the athlete truly loves the sport in question. When an athlete volitionally engages in sport because she values the benefits that are derived from participation, then this athlete is also autonomously motivated. Contemporary theories of motivation and research indicate that more autonomous motivation is "quality" motivation. Athletes who have quality motivation are more likely to work hard and work effectively, and their sense of who they are as people (i.e., their self-worth) is less tied to their sport performance. They tend to "keep on going," even when all is not going well and the extrinsic rewards associated with sport engagement are diminished or no longer exist. Autonomous motivation is predictive of greater sport enjoyment, feelings of vitality, and the tendency to define success in terms of doing one's best.

However, there are nonautonomous reasons for engaging in sport that are indicative of low quality motivation. Some athletes feel "controlled" in terms of why they are participating. They may be involved out of feelings of guilt or coercion; for example, they think they will let someone down (e.g., the coach, their parents) if they quit. Athletes can also participate in sport primarily because of extrinsic reasons (e.g., notoriety, accolades, and financial reward). In either case, someone or something else is "pulling the strings" in regard to reasons for engaging in sport. Controlled motivation is associated with heightened anxiety and a propensity for burnout, fear of failure, contingent self-worth, and intentions to drop out of sport (Figure 3.1).

REASONS FOR SPORT ENGAGEMENT

CONTROLLED MOTIVATION

AUTONOMOUS MOTIVATION

- EXTRINSIC REWARDS AND REINFORCEMENTS (MATERIAL, SOCIAL)

- COERCION
- INTERNALISED PRESSURE TO PARTICIPATE

- PERSONALLY VALUED BENEFITS

- INTRINSIC LOVE OF SPORT
- PARTICIPATES OUT OF PERSONAL CHOICE

NEGATIVE OUTCOMES

POSITIVE OUTCOMES

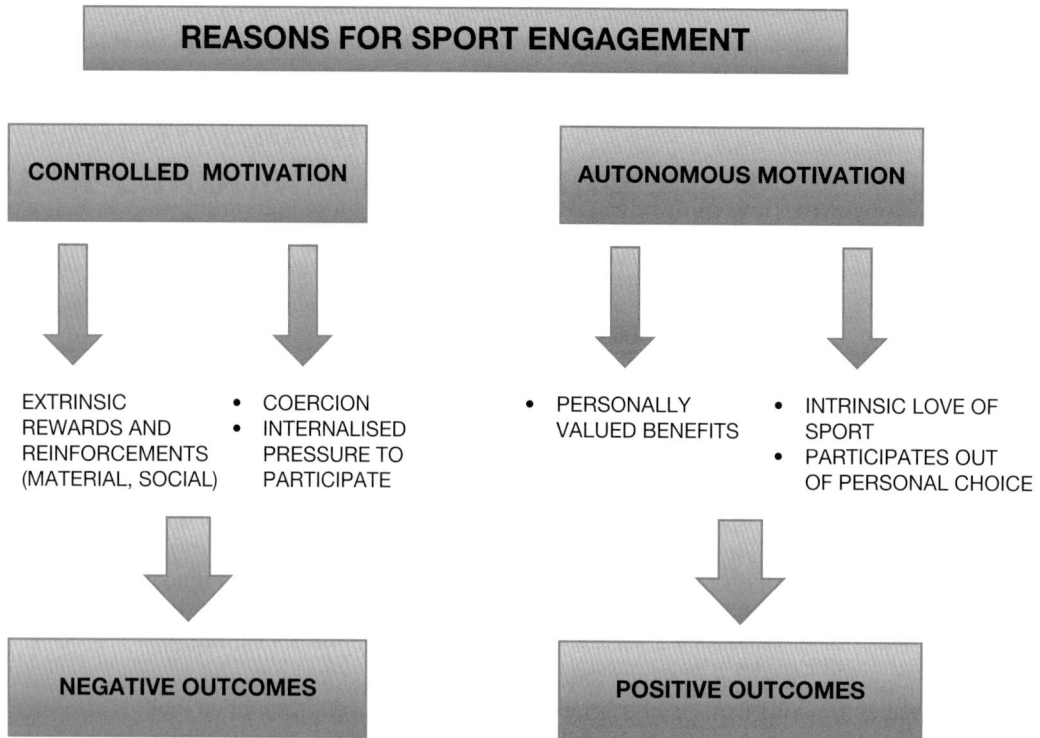

Figure 3.1 Autonomous and controlled reasons for engagement and their implications for positive/negative outcomes in sport

The coach-created environment and athletes' motivation

A key determinant of whether athletes are likely to exhibit autonomous and/or controlled motivation is the social psychological environment (or motivational climate) created by the coach. Theories of motivation and related research indicate which types of environments are more conducive to quality engagement and which coach behaviors are more likely to lead to controlled reasons for engagement.

One important feature of a coach-created environment, which holds significance for athletes' motivation, is the degree to which it is marked by autonomy support. In essence, autonomy support nurtures and maintains autonomous motivation. Coaches who are autonomy supportive (i) provide their athletes with meaningful choices and solicit their input, (ii) acknowledge the perspective of their athletes, (iii) minimize the use of extrinsic reward and when present, do not use them to control their athletes, and (iv) offer a rationale for requests and recommendations made.

Quality or more autonomous motivation is also facilitated when coaches are more task-involving. Task-involving coach behaviors include emphasizing when athletes try hard and exhibit learning and/or performance improvement. Socially supportive coaches also contribute to athletes' autonomous reasons for sport engagement. A socially supportive coach is one who cares, is there to help when needed, and separates the athlete from the performance.

Recently in the literature, autonomy supportive, task-involving and socially supportive coach behaviors have been conceptualized as the building blocks to a more "empowering" climate. In an empowering climate, athletes have a sense of ownership over their engagement and are "free" to grow and develop optimally in and through their sport. An "empowering" climate brings out the best in athletes, whether they are high in confidence or struggling with performance slumps, injury, or some other issue that is negatively impacting their perceptions of ability.

Coaches can also exhibit more "disempowering" behaviors that encourage controlled motivation in their athletes. Controlling coaches (i) employ intimidation, (ii) use extrinsic rewards to manipulate athletes to do what they want, (iii) engage in punitive actions, (iv) are authoritarian, and (v) show athletes that their approval is depending on the athlete being compliant and performing well. Ego-involving behaviors by the coach also contribute to a "disempowering" climate and evoke controlled motivation. In an ego-involving environment, coaches emphasize the importance of being the best (showing superiority) over doing one's best and make it apparent which athletes are considered more able or talented in their eyes. These are the type of coaches for whom "winning is everything and the only thing" with the athletes' development and welfare considered less important.

Research has shown that more disempowering coach-created motivational climates are linked to greater anxiety, lower morale functioning (e.g., as evidenced by cheating), and intentions to drop out. The negative impact of such environments is particularly marked on an athlete who is low in confidence. This finding is of particular relevance to female athletes, who are still more likely to doubt their abilities and have a more fragile sense of self than their male counterparts (Figure 3.2).

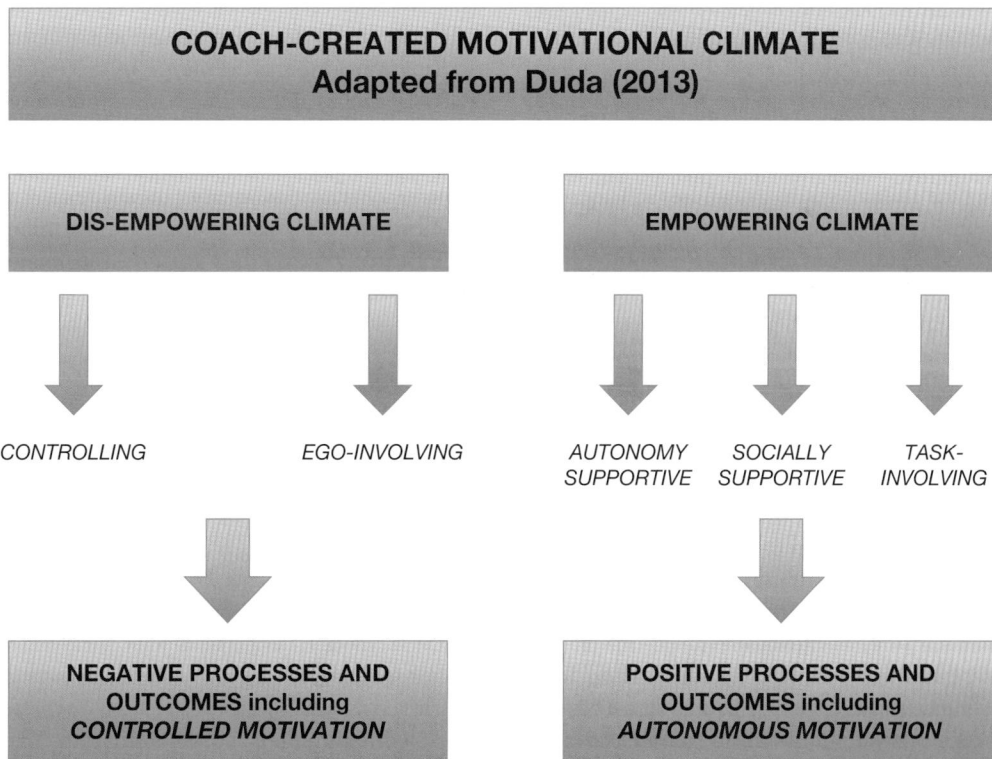

Figure 3.2 Dimensions and implications of 'empowering' and 'dis-empowering' climates as conceptualised by Duda (2013)

Training to change the motivational climate

Recent research in sport psychology has indicated that coaches can be trained up to be more empowering/less disempowering. Such a training program entails having coaches understand the how and why of an empowering approach and also become more cognizant of the costs of disempowering environments on athletes' health and well-being, development, and sustained engagement.

The literature also points to the relevance of other people besides the coach on the quality of motivation exhibited by athletes. There are numerous people who play a role in forming the climate that surrounds athletes, such as their parents, teammates, the National Governing Body or sport organization itself, and the members of the sport medicine team and other health care providers who work with them. It would be advantageous for all of these "significant others" to be educated on how they can be more autonomy supportive, task-involving, and socially supportive during their interactions. It is important as well that such relevant others in athletes' lives are informed, so they can recognize their disempowering behaviors and have the tools to change.

The female athlete and mental health issues/disorders

Recent research shows that the prevalence of mental health issues in elite athletes to be as high, if not higher, than in the normal population. In the past, it was believed that because athletes are, "emotionally very strong people", mental disorders did not exist in athletes at the elite level. A recent study showed that anxiety disorders and depression are the most common psychiatric disorders seen in the female athlete (including obsessive-compulsive disorder). Other diagnoses and mental health issues seen in the female athlete include attention deficit hyperactivity disorder (ADHD), eating disorders/female athlete triad along with issues involving substance abuse, the use of performance-enhancing drugs, retirement, abnormal or arrested development of life skills, child and adolescent issues, and difficulties with sexual harassment and abuse in sport (www.olympic.org/sha). Lastly, aggression or lack of aggression and self-confidence issues can also cause challenges for the female athlete.

Primary goals of sport psychiatry

To truly understand sport psychiatry, one must know what a sport psychiatrist qualifications are and what he or she can offer an elite female athlete that is novel and progressive. A sport psychiatrist is a physician who has specialized in psychiatry. They also have an expertise of all common psychiatric disorders in elite athletes and how to diagnose them. This allows for the most advantageous treatment of problems and symptoms, with the fewest side effects to the athlete. It also offers a better understanding of the difficulties the athlete is facing, with the athletes consent, by communication to the coach, their teammates, their family, and other significant others. Sport psychiatrists also have an understanding of the WADA Prohibited Substance List, how to manage the antidoping therapeutic use exemption (TUE) system, an athlete's fear of taking medication, and although decreasing as time moves forward, the stigmatization and possible ostracizing by teammates of seeing a psychiatrist.

The primary aims of the specialty are to (i) optimize physical and mental health, (ii) ethically improve athletic performance including optimizing coping mechanisms and positive psychological strengths, and (iii) manage psychiatric symptoms or disorders. This is different from both general internal medicine and from psychology. Once a diagnosis is made, the sport psychiatrist has a myriad of treatment options. Treatments can be optimized for the female athlete to experience the least side effects from medication that can be found in evidence-based scientific literature. For many athletes and coaches, medication can be seen as a treatment of last resort, which is understandable considering their side effects and that other treatments are increasingly available. Psychotherapies such as supportive, cognitive behavioral, analytic, and mindfulness-based stress reduction are available both individually and with groups and families. Mindfulness-based stress reduction groups utilize visualization, imagery, yoga, and the mind to control emotional reactions and "step back" so that the athlete can better understand her feelings. Performance-enhancing techniques and strategies, substance abuse/dependence management and treatment, MST, and self-help groups are also available.

Common psychiatric disorders in female athletes

By far and away, the anxiety and mood disorders are the most common psychiatric disorders seen in all athletes. In general, females are twice as likely to suffer from the anxiety disorders and have a slightly higher rate of obsessive compulsive disorder then males in adolescence and adulthood.

Anxiety disorders

The most common mental health issues and psychiatric disorders seen in female athletes are those related to anxiety. For the female athlete, it is almost impossible to have a normal life outside of sport. The female athlete is always extremely busy with her sport. They are always engaged in training and constantly travelling which make having meaningful intimate relationships and raising and nurturing children very challenging. It is important for the athlete, coach, or other members of the athlete entourage, to recognize rapidly increasing anxiety symptoms as early as possible, because an athlete can become debilitated by their anxiety. Stress and anxiety are an inherent part of sport. How an athlete deals with anxiety and stress can be the difference between gold and silver. But when a female athlete has either poor coping mechanisms to deal with her anxiety or the mounting numbers of stressors are such that anyone would become

incapacitated with anxiety, one must be alert that an athlete is not suffering from an anxiety disorder.

Common anxiety disorders in the female athlete

First, generalized anxiety disorder occurs when a female athlete has an increased level of anxiety over multiple issues; many of which, on their own, would not normally bring on heightened anxiety. The athlete's ability to perform well at her sport decreases because of this increased anxiety. The athlete can be tremulous, sweaty, have an increased heart and respiratory rate, feel nauseated, overwhelmed, and have a sense of impending doom. Second, one can see a spectrum of everything from obsessive-compulsive disorder to obsessive personality traits to ritualistic behaviors in athletes who are experiencing a generalized anxiety disorder. Almost all athletes have rituals. The more anxious one becomes, the more ritualistic behaviors increase. As this occurs, the female athlete can become more obsessive and perfectionist, which can detract from her ability to effectively concentrate and perform optimally. In the most severe cases, this can go onto a full-blown obsessive-compulsive disorder.

Lastly, acute stress disorder and posttraumatic stress disorder, now listed in a new category of disorders in the recently published Diagnostic and Statistical Manual, 5th edn (DSM-5), can occur in athletes. If the female athlete has a history of rape or is being sexually harassed and/or abused or the athlete has had a "traumatic" injury, she may be psychologically traumatized. The female athlete may start having nightmares, an increase in startle response, and extreme fear of the area where the rape or accident occurred amongst other physical and mental symptoms of anxiety, even horror. She may become extremely traumatized every time she is near the perpetrator of the abuse or rape or situation where the injury took place. The female athlete is twice as likely to be sexually harassed and/or abused in sport than their male counterparts while males are more likely to be the perpetrator. It is important to recognize that a psychologically traumatic personal event can bring on stress- and trauma-related disorders in athletes as in anyone in the normal population.

Mood disorders

Depression is one of the most common psychological problems encountered by athletes. Females experience a 1.5- to 3-fold higher rate than males of experiencing a major depressive episode beginning in early adolescence. Being a female with mental illness can create a double burden of discrimination. The stigma surrounding the use of psychiatric services can play a discouraging role in the athlete's illness and/or her injury recovery process. Sometimes coaches have difficulties looking past the physical difficulty leaving athletes' mental health issues untreated.

There are six times during an athlete's career when she is at particular risk of developing depressive symptoms or a major depressive episode. An athlete can suffer from depression for the same reasons as anyone in the normal population (e.g., the loss of a loved one). There is a clear link between concussions and new onset of clinical depression. Overtraining can also lead to athletic burnout and depression. Exercise and athletic training can be used as a defence against underlying issue/issues which can lead to depression. By throwing all one's emotional energy into elite sport, one can put off many of other life's psychological challenges. Difficult life transitions due to injury in sport or impending retirement can bring on depressive symptoms in elite female athletes. The signs and symptoms of clinical depression can be found in Table 3.1.

Table 3.1 Signs and symptoms of major depression

- Mood—sad, irritable
- Loss of interest (anhedonia)
- Change in appetite
- Change in sleep habits
- Decreased concentration
- Guilt
- Hopelessness, helplessness
- Loss of libido
- Loss of energy
- Suicidal ideation and/or attempt

Treatment for anxiety and mood disorders

The psychotherapies are the least intrusive treatments for anxiety and mood disorders. Supportive psychotherapy can be done by anyone within the athlete entourage. Supportive psychotherapy involves "being there" for the female athlete in an unconditional manner. The person engaged with the athlete in supportive psychological ways can do much to help the athlete during the acute phase or early stages of mental health issues. This is especially important in the female athlete who is used to being the nurturer rather than allowing others to nurture her. Cognitive-behavioral therapy is a well-proven therapy that helps the athlete or patient see life from a more positive position, one that does not put the blame on them. Analytic psychotherapy may be necessary when mental health issues are more ingrained, causing a repetitious pattern of behavior, such as choking in a competition while always succeeding in practice. Mindfulness-based stress reduction therapy is a recent, very popular therapy. It involves having the athlete or patient to look inward when they have intense feelings. Rather than "reacting," the athlete needs to try and step back and understand and analyze their feelings. The aim is to see how their enhanced "Mindfulness" can help with a healthier response by using yoga, relaxation techniques, visualization and imagery to decrease the anxiety and depressive feelings.

A sport psychiatrist can prescribe medications if necessary. The antidepressant and anti-anxiety antidepressants are not on the WADA Prohibited Substance List. The sport psychiatrist understands the sport culture and an athlete's possible initial reluctance to take medication. Many of the medications that would be used to treat anxiety and mood disorders have similar mechanisms of action and are from similar classes of drugs. They are not addictive; however, as with all medications, they may have side effects. The sport psychiatrist must work with the female athlete to ensure that the medications used have the least possible number of side effects, especially side effects that can affect performance. It is also important to mention that no matter what the treatment used for any mental health issue, the earlier it is recognized, the more likely the athlete will recover from any difficulties that they were having initially

Female athlete triad/disordered eating and eating disorder

For many years, psychiatry has looked at female patients with disordered eating and the physical and mental sequelae that follow such restrictive or irregular eating habits as suffering from an "eating disorder." In the normal population, females are ten times more likely to develop an eating disorder as compared to men, with a prevalence rate of 0.4% in a 12-month period. Within the world of sport, the "at-risk sports" for disordered eating are those sports in which body weight can affect performance outcome; the aesthetic sports, sports with body weight classes, and those sports in which low weight can give an advantage, such as marathon running. The female athlete, coach, and athlete entourage all need to be aware of signs and symptoms of disordered eating to try and revert to healthy and nutritious dietary practices before the athlete needs treatment for a full-blown eating disorder.

In parallel, but specific to the world of sport, a body of scientific literature that considers disordered eating and its health implications continues to grow on what is known as "the female athlete triad" or just "the triad." The triad consists of three physiological components in female athletes: energy availability, menstrual functioning, and bone density or health. When discussing the triad, if female athletes' energy intake is deficient (in regard to calories consumed) via a purposeful and desirable (in terms of performance as well as her health) decrease in intake and an increase in exercise, this can simply be referred to as a weight-reduction diet. Unfortunately, inadequate energy intake can also occur in the female athlete without her knowledge because of an increase in training without an increase in energy input, leading to insufficient energy intake, menstrual irregularities, such as oligomenorrhea, amenorrhea, and other

such menstrual cycle irregularities and decreased bone density. This can lead to a series of detrimental physical and mental consequences and obviously, if not immediate, then eventual poor performance outcomes. Initially one sees increased protein retention, decreased energy intake, and the early stages of kidney disease. Decreased energy intake can also cause decreased concentration and mood irritability and depression, along with menstrual abnormalities and decrease in bone density, as seen in the "triad."

If energy intake continues to decrease, the female athlete can unfortunately begin suffering from one or more of the eating disorders, as defined by the psychiatric DSM-5. The eating disorders include anorexia nervosa, bulimia nervosa, binge eating disorder, and other specified (or unspecified) feeding or eating disorder. Anorexia nervosa and bulimia nervosa affect mainly young women. Anorexia nervosa can be described as a pathological fear of becoming fat combined with a distorted body image. The female athlete is led to excessive dieting followed by an unhealthy weight loss. Bulimia nervosa is characterized by periods of binge eating followed by purging behaviors such as self-induced vomiting, excessive exercise, and use of laxatives (or other medications). In the case of a binge eating disorder, one sees recurrent episodes of eating large amounts of food in short bursts of time combined with shame, guilt, and feelings of a lack of control while the binge is occurring. DSM-5 has one last category of eating disorders, namely "otherwise specified" or "unspecified." This category includes all disordered eating behaviors that cause psychological distress and functional impairment not fitting the criteria of one of the other eating disorders. Starvation, such as seen in anorexia, causes profound weight loss, hypothermia, low heart rate, hypotension, lanugo (soft fuzzy hair on the body), cardiac abnormalities, and gastric dilation. Purging behaviors such as the use of diuretics and laxatives can lower potassium leading to renal failure and cardiac arrest. Such purging behaviors can cause esophageal tears from vomiting or attempted vomiting and dental carries and poor dentition can occur from acid reflux from the stomach. One can also see swollen salivary glands on the face. The earlier a female athlete seeks treatment for their

Table 3.2   How to approach the female athlete with disordered eating behavior?

1. **Direct and empathic approach**—Discuss in a private and quiet place without interruption. Tell the athlete you are worried about her and why (e.g., teammates have seen you vomiting after meals).
2. **Avoid threats of manipulation**—Tell the athlete that she has a problem and it is her problem not your problem. Indicate that you will help the athlete get assistance if she needs it. Stand your ground firmly and compassionately.
3. **If the athlete refuses help**—If there are enough reasons to be concerned, a coach or parent should consider removing the athlete from the sport until she seeks help. This could be a lifesaving intervention.

disordered eating or eating disorder, the faster the recovery. Since eating disorders and disordered eating cause increased morbidity and even mortality, it is imperative that the coach and the entire athlete entourage are hypervigilant in early recognition, discussion of the issue with the athlete (see Table 3.2), and seek professional help as soon as possible.

Attention deficit hyperactive disorder (ADHD)

ADHD is a neurodevelopmental disorder that causes inattention, disorganization, and/or hyperactivity-impulsivity. Inattention and disorganization can be seen by an inability to stay on task, seeming not to listen, and losing or misplacing materials, at levels that are inconsistent with the age or developmental level of the athlete in question. Hyperactivity-impulsivity includes behaviors such as constant activity, fidgeting, inability to stay seated, intruding into other people's activities, and inability to wait. ADHD is two times more likely to be seen in the child male athlete when compared to the young female athlete and that ratio (female/male) is 1.6:1 in adults. Globally, ADHD is a controversial diagnosis, as some countries do not believe the disorder exists. In North America, ADHD is the most common reason for the child/adolescent patient to be referred to mental health services. The treatment of choice for ADHD is one of the psycho-stimulants. Since the psycho-stimulants are on the WADA Prohibited Substance List, the female athlete must apply for a TUE. As such, the athlete must have proper documentation. The diagnostic assessment, along with regular assessments from diagnosis to the present, preferably from a psychologist or psychiatrist that has an expertise in this area, is the best course of action. Old report cards and parental accounts are also helpful, as to obtain a TUE for the psycho-stimulant, the athlete must prove that she has met the criteria to be diagnosed with the disorder according to DSM-5. One can see how a psychiatrist that specializes in sport would make this process easier. The sport psychiatrist would also be aware of any medical testing that the athlete, who is diagnosed with ADHD, may need and knows how to monitor the athlete to minimize side effects of any medication used.

Conclusion

The field of sport psychiatry tends to be an underutilized area in the world of sport. As mental health issues are certainly evident among elite competitors, there is a need for specialized psychiatric care to promote healthy functioning and combat psychologically grounded performance difficulties in the case of high-level athletes.

Not all the challenges facing talented athletes are clinical in nature, however. Moreover, just because an athlete is no longer experiencing angst or duress means that he or she is healthy and functioning well. The aspiration is to have elite athletes not just *survive* the demands and pressures of being a high-level competitor but also to *thrive* within the elite sport setting. It is important for sport psychologists and sport psychiatrists not only to address serious problems and complications that some athletes may face, but also to support *all* athletes in optimizing what they accomplish in sport, how they feel about their sport and feel about themselves when participating, and what the impact of sport engagement is on their lives...as athletes and as girls/women. The literature is clear that, via the creation of more "empowering" climates within the sport world, the promotion of more autonomous sport motivation, and the fostering of self-regulation abilities, female athletes are more likely to overcome their adversities and flourish. Moreover, if prevailing sporting environments were more "empowering" and less "disempowering," this would contribute to greater prevention of a number of the mental health issues faced by female athletes.

With these aspirations in mind, we argue that sport psychology and sport psychiatry are two complementary and necessary fields. Professionals who represent these two professional backgrounds share some methods and techniques but also offer different approaches and treatments. The inclusion of these two disciplinary perspectives will only strengthen research on the psychology of female athletes. When formulating sports medicine teams, it would be prudent to include practitioners representing each of these specializations.

Recommended reading

American Psychiatric Association. (2013) *Diagnostic and Statistical Manual of Mental Disorders* (5th edn). American Psychiatric Association, Washington, DC.

Balaguer I, González L, Fabra P, Castillo I, Mercé J, and Duda JL. (2012) Coaches' interpersonal style, basic psychological needs and the well- and ill-being of young soccer players: a longitudinal analysis. *J Sports Sci*, 30, 1619–1629.

Baron DI, Reardon CL, and Baron SH (eds). (2013) *Clinical Sports Psychiatry—An International Perspective*. Wiley-Blackwell, New York.

Begel D. (1992) An overview of sport psychiatry. *Am J Psychiatry*, 49, 606–614.

Conant-Norville DO and Tofler IR. (2005) Attention deficit/hyperactivity disorder and psychopharmacologic treatments in the athlete. *Clin Sports Med*, 24, 829–843.

Duda JL. (2013) The conceptual and empirical foundations of Empowering Coaching™: setting the stage for the PAPA Project. *Int J Spt Exer Psych*, 11(4), 311–318.

Duda JL and Balaguer I. (2007) The coach-created motivational climate. In SJowett and DLavalee (eds), *Social Psychology of Sport* (pp. 117–130). Human Kinetics, Champaign, IL.

Duda JL, Cumming J, and Balaguer I. (2005) Enhancing athletes' self regulation, task involvement, and self determination via psychological skills training. In DHackfort, JDuda, and RLider (eds), *Handbook of Applied Sport Psychology Research* (pp. 159–181). Fitness Information Technology, Morgantown, WV.

Durand-Bush N and Salmela JH. (2002) The development and maintenance of expert athletic performance: perceptions of World and Olympic champions. *J Appl Sport Psychol*, 14, 154–171.

Edenfield TM and Saeed SA. (2012) An update on mindfulness meditation as a self-help treatment for anxiety and depression. *Psychol Res Behav Management*, 5, 131–141.

Glick ID, Kamm R, and Morse E. (2009) The evolution of sport psychiatry, Circa 2009, *Sports Med*, 39(8), 607–613.

Kamm RL. (2005) Interviewing principles for the psychiatrically aware sports medicine physician. *Clin Sports Med*, 255, 745–769.

Marks SI, Mountjoy ML, and Marcus M. (2012) Sexual harassment and abuse in sport: the role of the team doctor. *British J Sports Med*, 46, 905–908.

Ryan RM and Deci EL. (2000) Self-determination theory and the facilitation of intrinsic motivation, social development, and well-being. *Am Psychol*, 55, 68–78.

Salmi M, Pichard C, and Jousselin E. (2010) Psychopathology and high level sport. *Sci and Sports*, 25, 1–10.

Sharp L-A, Woodcock C, Holland MJG, Cumming J, and Duda JL. (2013) A qualitative evaluation of the effectiveness of a mental skills training program for youth athletes. *Sport Psychol*, 27, 219–232.

Williams J and Krane V (eds). (2014) *Applied Sport Psychology: Personal Growth to Peak Performance* (7th edn). McGraw-Hill, New York.

Chapter 4
Nutritional guidelines for female athletes

Louise M. Burke

Sports Nutrition, Australian Institute of Sport, Belconnen, ACT, Australia

Introduction

Good nutrition is important for optimal performance for all athletes, but particularly so for females. Female athletes have increased requirements for some nutrients compared with males. In addition, due to their smaller body size and often a relative smaller training load, female athletes need to achieve their nutritional requirements from a smaller energy intake. Finally, female athletes in at least some sports appear to be at greater risk of developing issues related to eating and body image compared with their sedentary counterparts or male athletes. Therefore, there are some challenges but great rewards for achieving a sound eating plan. This chapter overviews the key concepts of sports nutrition considering whether the current guidelines are suitable for female athletes and providing special insights into issues that might be different to those of their male counterparts.

Specificity and periodization of nutrition goals

A variety of nutrition goals can be identified in the training and competition elements of sporting involvement (see Table 4.1). It is important to realize, however, that these goals and nutritional requirements are not only specific to the individual athlete and her event, but specific to the phase of the athlete's program. Athletes incorporate a range of training sessions (type, duration and intensity) within the microcycles and macrocycles of their conditioning programs, and compete in events with a range of different nutritional challenges. There are also differences in individual responses to many nutritional interventions, and a need to integrate the athlete's range of sports nutrition and other "everyday" or clinical nutrition goals into her overall eating program. Therefore, each athlete needs an individualized plan to achieve her unique set of nutrition goals and requirements and should expect that her eating plan will differ from day to day and over the season to accommodate changes in the exercise load and other goals of the periodized approach to conditioning and performance.

Can research on male athletes be applied to females?

Expert groups that develop sports nutrition guidelines typically make universal recommendations without specific adjustment for the sex of the individual athlete. The absence of sex-specific guidelines could mean that females do not have special considerations regarding exercise metabolism or nutritional requirements for sport. Alternatively, it could mean that there is no information on

The Female Athlete, First Edition. Edited by Margo L. Mountjoy.
© 2015 International Olympic Committee. Published 2015 by John Wiley & Sons, Inc.

Table 4.1 A summary of sports nutrition goals

In training, the athlete should aim to
- Meet the energy and fuel requirements needed to support her training program
- Achieve a physique (body mass, body fat, and muscle mass) that is consistent with long-term health and performance using sensible strategies
- Refuel and rehydrate well for key training sessions where it is important to perform at her best
- Enhance recovery and adaptation between training sessions by providing all the nutrients associated with these processes
- Practice any intended competition nutrition strategies so that beneficial practices can be identified and fine-tuned
- Reduce the risk of illness and injury during heavy training periods by maintaining healthy physique and energy balance and meeting requirements for key micronutrients (e.g., iron, calcium) and health-promoting food chemicals (e.g., antioxidants, omega fatty acids)

In competition, the athlete should aim to
- In weight-division sports, achieve the competition weight division with minimal harm to health or performance
- "Fuel up" adequately prior to an event; consume carbohydrate and achieve exercise taper during the day(s) prior to the event according to the importance and duration of the event; and utilize carbohydrate-loading strategies when appropriate before events of greater than 90-minute duration
- Use opportunities to drink before and during the event to minimize dehydration by replacing most of the sweat losses, but without drinking in excess of sweat losses
- Consume carbohydrates during events >1 hour in duration with a sliding scale of intake according to the need to prime the brain or to provide an additional source of muscle fuel.
- Achieve pre-event and during-event eating/drinking strategies without causing gastrointestinal discomfort or upsets
- Promote recovery after the event, particularly during multiday competitions such as tournaments and stage races

Overall
- Make use of supplements and specialized sports foods that have been shown to enhance training goals or provide a competition performance gain after considering the potential risks associated with their use
- Eat for long-term health by paying attention to community nutrition guidelines
- Continue to enjoy food and the pleasure of sharing meals

which the effect of sex can be based. It is of importance to differentiate between these two options since the absence of evidence for an effect is not the same as evidence for the absence of an effect. Three broad categories of studies would be useful in either confirming the suitability of present sports nutrition guidelines or developing separate recommendations for female athletes: (i) studies in which female subjects have been included within the group outcomes without distinguishing any differences based on sex; (ii) studies that focus on female subjects alone, and (iii) research in which direct comparisons have been made between the response of male and female subjects to a sports nutrition intervention. It is clear, notwithstanding the difficulties of undertaking such research, that these types of studies are under-represented in the literature and should be encouraged.

There are several issues that might explain or call for differences in recommendations for sports nutrition for female athletes. The first is the different hormonal environment and its changes over the menstrual cycle experienced by females. The small number of factors in which this has been investigated in terms of exercise metabolism (e.g., protein synthesis and carbohydrate metabolism) suggests that such differences, if they occur, are sufficiently subtle that they do not merit separate recommendations in terms of sports nutritional strategies. The second issue is the smaller body size or muscle mass of females. This issue is covered to some extent in that old sports nutrition recommendations for absolute nutrient amounts have been replaced with targets expressed relative to body mass (e.g., carbohydrate intake) or in terms of developing an individualized and tolerated plan (e.g., fluid intake during exercise). A final consideration is the observation that many female athletes consume diets that are low in energy availability; apart from impairing health and function, this can indirectly alter nutritional requirements.

Low energy availability

An inadequate intake of energy in relation to the energy cost of exercise prevents the body from having sufficient energy to fuel the functions underpinning optimal health and performance. This situation, termed low energy availability, is frequently observed among female athletes related to their management of optimal body mass/physique. However, it can also occur when appetite or opportunities to consume food fail to adapt to an increase in training/competition load. The chapter on the female athlete triad (Chapter 9) describes the causes and outcomes of this syndrome in more detail. Here, we will quickly consider the effects of low energy availability on sports nutrition requirements. Although the clear objective is for female athletes to avoid scenarios of energy deficiency, there are some situations in which some reduction in energy availability may be required or tolerated. In such cases, some secondary nutritional issues should be considered.

An outcome of the reduction in energy intake below energy expenditure is an adjustment to physiological function to conserve energy and preserve against starvation. A reduction in metabolic rate ultimately reduces energy requirements, whereby in extreme cases, a female may regain energy balance (intake = expenditure) despite a low level of energy availability (where EA = intake minus the energy cost of exercise < level required for healthy function). In these cases, nutritional counseling of the female athlete may need to take into account a current energy requirement below predicted/healthy levels. A gradual intake in energy may be required to help restore energy availability, metabolic rate, and health. Even when this takes place, however, the female athlete will need to make sound dietary choices from a range of nutrient-dense foods to ensure that all requirements for micronutrients and beneficial food constituents are met from a restricted energy budget. The case for reduced EA and the protein and carbohydrate guidelines covered later in this chapter merit special comment.

Older studies of female athletes and carbohydrate loading made observations that they are less efficient at storing glycogen than their male counterparts (i.e., females store less glycogen from a given carbohydrate intake or fail to supercompensate muscle glycogen stores). More recent research has shown that this finding is related to

energy deficiency and females can store glycogen effectively when they consume adequate energy intake. Alternatively, when carbohydrate intake is below the targets identified for optimal refueling, the addition of protein (~20 g) to the meal/snack enhances glycogen storage. Meanwhile, although protein targets can be set for meals and snacks to optimize protein synthesis in response to exercise over the day, recent studies show that these targets need to be increased even when energy availability is reduced by amounts normally considered to be "safe" for weight loss (30 kcal/kg fat-free mass).

Guidelines for everyday training

Everyday eating must support the athlete's training load and allow her to stay healthy and uninjured. The fuel cost of training varies according to the frequency, duration, and intensity of workouts, and causes a change in the athlete's daily carbohydrate use. Sports nutrition guidelines have changed from recommending that all athletes consume "high carbohydrate diets" per se to considering carbohydrate intake in relation to the fuel cost of training and refueling ("carbohydrate availability"). The guidelines recommend that for days/scenarios where the training program calls for high-intensity, high-quality or technique-based workouts, athletes should consume carbohydrate over the day and in relation to the workout to provide high carbohydrate availability (carbohydrate targets met). General targets have been set (Table 4.2) but need to be individualized according to the athlete, her energy budget, and feedback from training outcomes and long-term performance gains. Meanwhile, in other scenarios, carbohydrate availability may not be crucial for training outcomes, and the athlete can allow carbohydrate intake to be below theoretical exercise costs. In fact, there are even potential advantages to periodizing training to include some sessions involving low carbohydrate availability (training after an overnight fast, training with low glycogen stores, etc.) to promote a greater training stimulatory response.

Muscle protein synthesis is a desired response to an exercise session, with the specific stimulus

Table 4.2 Carbohydrate intake targets for athletes

	Situation	Carbohydrate targets	Comments on type and timing of carbohydrate intake
DAILY NEEDS FOR FUEL AND RECOVERY—these general recommendations should be fine-tuned with individual consideration of total energy needs, specific training needs, and feedback from training performance			
Light	• Low intensity or skill-based activities	3–5 g/kg of athlete's body mass/day	• Timing of intake may be chosen to promote speedy refueling or to provide fuel intake around training sessions in the day. Otherwise, as long as total fuel needs are provided, the pattern of intake may simply be guided by convenience and individual choice
Moderate	• Moderate exercise program (i.e., ~1 h/day)	5–7 g/kg/day	
High	• Endurance program (e.g., 1–3 h/day mod-high intensity exercise)	6–10 g/kg/day	• Protein and nutrient-rich carbohydrate food or food combinations will allow the athlete to meet other acute or chronic sports nutrition goals
Very high	• Extreme commitment (i.e., >4–5 h/day mod-high intensity exercise	8–12 g/kg/day	
ACUTE FUELING STRATEGIES—these guidelines promote high carbohydrate availability to promote optimal performance in competition or key training sessions			
General fuelling up	• Preparation for events < 90 minutes exercise	7–12 g/kg per 24 hours as for daily fuel needs	• Athletes may choose compact carbohydrate-rich sources that are low in fiber/residue and easily consumed to ensure that fuel targets are met, and to meet goals for gut comfort or lighter "racing weight"
Carbohydrate loading	• Preparation for events >90 minutes of sustained/intermittent exercise	36–48 hours of 10–12 g/kg per 24 hours	
Speedy refueling	• <8 hours recovery between 2 fuel demanding sessions	1–1.2 g/kg/h for first 4 hours then resume daily fuel needs	• There may be benefits in consuming small regular snacks • Compact carbohydrate-rich food and drinks may help to ensure that fuel targets are met
Pre-event fuelling	• Before exercise (>60 minutes)	1–4 g/kg consumed 1–4 hours before exercise	• Timing, amount and type of carbohydrate food and drinks should suit the practical needs of the event, and individual preferences/experiences • Choices high in fat/protein/fiber may need to be avoided to reduce risk of gastrointestinal issues during the event • Low glycemic index choices may provide a more sustained source of fuel for situations where carbohydrate cannot be consumed during exercise
During brief exercise	• <45 minutes	Not needed	
During sustained high intensity exercise	• 45–75 minutes	Small amounts including mouth rinse	• A range of drinks and sports products can provide easily consumed carbohydrate
During endurance exercise including "stop and start" sports	• 1–2.5 hours	30–60 g/h	• Opportunities to consume food and drinks vary according to the rules and nature of each sport • A range of everyday dietary choices and specialized sports products ranging in form from liquid to solid may be useful • The athlete should practice to find a refueling plan that suits her individual goals including hydration needs and gut comfort
During ultra-endurance exercise	• >2.5–3 hours	Up to 90 g/h	• As above • Higher intakes of carbohydrate are associated with better performance • Products providing multiple transportable carbohydrates (glucose/fructose mixtures) will achieve high rates of oxidation of carbohydrate consumed during exercise

Source: Reprinted with permission from Burke *et al.* (2011).

of training targeting specific increases in protein types. There is a greater increase in myofibrillar proteins in response to resistance training, while endurance athletes are interested in an increase in the mitochondrial or sarcolemmal proteins that underpin metabolic goals. Insights from the latest protein research have moved guidelines away from a focus on over daily protein intake targets or the concept of nitrogen balance, to targets for chronically maximizing the protein synthetic response to training or competition. Although the period immediately after key exercise sessions is an important time to consume protein for this purpose, it is also important to consume protein over the next 24–48 hours to take advantage of the long stimulatory response to a workout. The new guidelines promote an intake of ~20 g (perhaps 15–30 g depending on body size, with the high-end of this range being required when in lower energy availability) of high-quality protein soon after exercise and at meals/snacks every 3–4 hours over the day. A protein-rich snack prior to bed will also assist with overnight protein synthesis. Lean meats, eggs, and low-fat dairy products provide a good source of such protein, as well as other micronutrients such as iron and calcium that can be in short supply in the diets of many female athletes. Vegetarian protein sources (e.g., soy milk, tofu, beans, and lentils) are typically limiting in some of the essential amino acids, but mixing and matching these sources together, or adding dairy or eggs in the case of lacto-ovo-vegetarians, will enhance the protein quality of the meal.

Calcium and vitamin D are micronutrients of major importance for bone health, although vitamin D is also involved in a variety of other activities such as immune health and muscle function. Unfortunately, many female athletes suffer from suboptimal status of these nutrients, which, when combined with the effects of low energy availability, can lead to poor bone health and its short-term (career-affecting injury) and long-term (increased risk of osteoporosis). In the case of calcium, adequacy of intake of dairy or fortified-soy products is the essential key strategy, while for vitamin D, there is a choice of safe sunshine exposure during periods in which UVB radiation is appropriate and/or vitamin D supplementation. Female

athletes who are at risk of inadequate UVB exposure (e.g., athletes from higher latitudes, those who have dark skin pigmentation or those who spend most of their time and training activities indoors) should be screened for vitamin D status and treated by appropriate experts. Athletes within any of the risks or issues of the female athlete triad should receive early assessment and intervention since the effects can be life-lasting (see Chapter 9).

Iron status is often also suboptimal in female athletes due to the combination of increased requirements (e.g., losses via menstruation) and poor intake of bioavailable iron (low intake of heme sources of iron or reduced absorption of iron due to the effects of exercise on the iron regulating hormone hepcidin). Iron deficiency anemia causes a clear impairment of performance, but even low iron status without anemia may cause fatigue and interfere with an athlete's ability to respond optimally to hard training. Female athletes at risk of poor iron status should have it checked and may need iron supplementation therapy as well as dietary advice to improve their dietary iron intake. It can be difficult for many female athletes to integrate all their dietary needs into a single eating plan that suits their energy and financial budgets, as well as their busy schedule of training, travel, and competition. The expertise of a sports nutritionist/dietitian can assist in developing a practical plan that is suitably individualized. Some of the food choices and eating strategies that allow multiple nutritional goals to be met simultaneously are summarized in Table 4.3.

Goals for altering physique

In a number of sports, physique characteristics play a direct role in performance. For example, a high-level of muscularity is favorable for activities based on strength and power. Low body mass and low levels of body fat are of value in sports where an athlete must move her body over a distance (e.g., distance running), against gravity (e.g., road cycling on a hilly course), or in a small space (e.g., gymnastics or diving). In other sports, athletes compete in weight divisions (e.g., boxing, lightweight rowing) or are judged on the aesthetics of their physique (e.g., bodybuilding, gymnastics).

Table 4.3 Characteristics of foods and food combinations which may be of particular value in menus for female athletes

Issue	Feature	Comments	Examples
Achieving targets for high-quality protein over the day	Postexercise	15–25 g of quickly digested leucine-rich protein after exercise will promote muscle protein synthesis	15 g of protein can be found in • 400 mL low-fat milk • 1 tub Greek yoghurt • 250 mL fortified milkshake or liquid meal/ protein supplement
	Meals and snacks	15–25 g of high-quality protein will continue to promote muscle protein synthesis over the day	15 g of protein can be found in • ~50–80 g lean meat/fish/chicken • 2 large or 3 small eggs • 60 g cheese
Achieving carbohydrate and nutrient requirements from a lower energy requirement (compared with males) or achieving weight management goals	Low-fat content	A low or reduced fat content reduces the energy content of the food/ meal supplying a targeted amount of carbohydrate.	• Low-fat flavored milk or yoghurt • Wholegrain cereal and low-fat milk • Wholegrain bread • Rice or pasta
	Low energy density/high satiety (fullness causing end of meal)	High water and fiber content allows a large volume of food to be consumed to provide a targeted carbohydrate serve.	• Fresh fruit • Thick vegetable soup and bread • Sandwich with thick salad filling • High vegetable content stir fry or casserole with noodles/rice
	Enhanced satiety (reduced hunger until next meal)	Low glycemic index carbohydrate choices may increase satiety. Co-ingestion of protein also increases the satiety of meals or snacks (see section below regarding protein).	• Rolled oats—porridge or Bircher muesli • Multigrained or sour dough breads • Sweetened dairy products • Baked beans on toast • Lentil curry/casserole • Noodles/pasta/quinoa/Basmati rice
	High nutrient density	Valuable source of high-quality protein in addition to carbohydrate content	• Low-fat sweetened yoghurt • Wholegrain cereal and low-fat milk • Eggs on toast
		Valuable source of iron in addition to carbohydrate content	• Sandwich with lean beef filling • Pasta with lean beef bolognaise sauce
		Valuable source of calcium in addition to carbohydrate content	• Low-fat sweetened yoghurt • Wholegrain cereal and low-fat milk • Reduced fat cheese on a pizza
		Valuable source of antioxidants in addition to carbohydrate content	• Fresh fruit • Thick vegetable soup and bread • Dried fruit and nut mix (almonds/walnuts)
Enhanced food enjoyment	Social eating opportunities	Many females enjoy the opportunity to consume meals and snacks in a special surrounding or a social eating situation rather than consuming energy simply to meet a specific nutritional goal.	• Skimmed milk hot chocolate or frappe drink in a cafe • Muffin or fruit bread in a cafe • Dessert in a restaurant

(continued)

Table 4.3 *(Continued)*

Issue	Feature	Comments	Examples
Enhanced food enjoyment *(continued)*	Observed preferences	Many female athletes appear to prefer sweet forms of carbohydrate in preference to savory carbohydrate-rich choices. They also prefer solid forms of carbohydrate to carbohydrate-rich fluids (e.g., sodas, sports drinks). The exception to this may be chocolate-flavored milk, but this is also preferred as a hot drink or a frozen drink (frappe), especially when consumed in a social setting (see above).	• Confectionery or sports confectionery (and water) instead of sports drinks during exercise • Low-fat dairy food rather than protein supplement for postexercise recovery • Low-fat sweetened yoghurt or dairy dessert (e.g., custard or fromage frais) rather than flavored milk • Carbohydrate-moderated main meal plus CHO-rich dessert rather than carbohydrate-rich main meal (e.g., pasta/rice dominated meal) • "Diet soda" and carbohydrate-rich snack rather than sweetened sodas

Some high-level athletes "naturally" display the physique characteristics that are required for their sport—as a result of the genetic traits that have caused them to gravitate to this activity as well as the conditioning effects of serious training. By contrast, other athletes have to undertake specific programs to manipulate their body mass, muscle mass, and body fat levels. In fact, weight loss is the most popular reason for a female athlete to consult a sports dietitian.

Many athletes pursue rigid criteria for the "ideal physique" for their sport, based on the characteristics of successful competitors, or in the case of sports-favoring leanness, the attainment of minimum levels of body fat. The pressure to conform to such an ideal comes from coaches, trainers, other athletes, as well as the athlete's own perfectionism and drive to succeed. However, there are several dangers and disadvantages to the establishment of rigid prescriptions for the body weight or body fat levels of individual athletes. First, it fails to acknowledge that there is a considerable variability in the physical characteristics of successful athletes, even between individuals in the same sport. It also fails to take into account that it can take many years of training and maturation for an athlete to finally achieve their ideal shape and body composition. Finally, it fails to realize that successful athletes periodize their physique so that their light/lean "race weights" are achieved only for short and specific periods of competition.

In any case, weight/fat loss should be achieved using targets that are achievable and with a pattern of gentle and sustained loss that still allows a dietary plan with sufficient energy availability, nutrient adequacy, and social enjoyment of food. Although it is difficult to get reliable figures on the prevalence of eating disorders or disordered eating behavior and body image among athletes, there appears to be a higher risk of problems among female athletes, particularly in sports in which success is associated with specific weight targets or low body fat levels. Even where clinical eating disorders do not exist, many female athletes appear to be "restrained eaters," reporting low energy intakes that are considerably less than expected energy requirements and considerable stress related to food intake. Expert advice from sports medicine professionals, including dietitians, psychologists, and physicians, is important in the early detection and management of problems related to body composition and nutrition (see Chapter 9).

An increase in muscle mass is desired by female athletes whose performance is linked with size, strength, or power (e.g., team athletes, weight lifters, rowers). These athletes pursue specific muscle hypertrophy through a program of progressive muscle overload. The important nutritional requirements to support such a program are adequate energy, and careful spacing of high-quality protein intake at meals and snacks after resistance workouts and over the day. Some female athletes do not achieve a sufficiently positive energy balance to optimize muscle gains during a strength-training program. Specialized nutrition advice can help the athlete improve this situation by making energy-dense foods and drinks accessible and easy to consume.

Guidelines for competition nutrition— fuelling up

During most competition activities, an athlete will experience deterioration in speed, power, skill, or the other attributes that define success in her event. To achieve optimal performance, she should identify potentially preventable factors that contribute to this fatigue and undertake nutritional strategies before, during, and after the event that minimize or delay its onset. This is obviously important during competition, but athletes should also practice such strategies during key training sessions, both to support technique and intensity during the workout and to fine-tune the nutritional plan for a specific event. The nutritional challenges of competition vary according to length and intensity of the event, the environment, and factors that influence the recovery between events or the opportunity to eat and drink during the event itself.

Carbohydrate availability for the muscle and central nervous system limits the performance of prolonged (>90 minutes) submaximal or intermittent high-intensity exercise. It also plays a permissive role in the performance of shorter high-intensity events. Competition eating should target strategies to consume carbohydrate before, during, or between such events to provide high carbohydrate availability. Carbohydrate should be consumed over the day(s) leading up to an event according to the muscle glycogen requirements of the task. The trained muscle is able to normalize its high resting stores with as little as 24 hours of rest and adequate intakes of carbohydrate (and energy) intake (see Table 4.2). Extending the time and carbohydrate ingestion to ~48 hours can achieve a super-compensation of muscle glycogen commonly known as carbohydrate loading. Such loading is important for events of more than 90-minute duration (e.g., marathons, Ironman triathlons). Carbohydrate eaten in the hours prior to an event can also ensure adequate liver glycogen, especially for events undertaken after an overnight fast. Although general recommendations can be provided for the pre-event meal (Table 4.2), the type, timing, and amount of carbohydrate-rich foods and drinks will need to be chosen with consideration of practical issues such as gastrointestinal comfort, individual preferences, and catering arrangements in the competition environment. The athlete should practice with her precompetition eating to develop an individualised plan.

Fuelling and hydrating during competitions

In sporting activities of greater than 45 minutes, there is usually an opportunity and a benefit from consuming nutrients during the event. During sporting activities lasting longer than ~75 minutes, there is good evidence that carbohydrate consumed during the event can supply an additional source of fuel for the muscle to enhance performance. For events of up to about 2–2.5h, an intake of ~30–60 g of carbohydrate per hour appears to be a suitable target. However, for activities of longer duration (e.g., marathons, cycling stage races, Ironman triathlon), recent research has suggested that even higher rates of carbohydrate intake (e.g., up to 80–90 g/h) achieve greater benefits. The previous guidelines were mindful that intestinal absorption of carbohydrate during exercise limited the exogenous supply of carbohydrate to the working muscle to about 60 g/h. However, it now appears that this limitation can be overcome by consuming a mixture of carbohydrate sources that use different intestinal transport mechanisms, such as fructose and glucose. Such mixes permit higher rates of oxidation of ingested carbohydrate and better gastrointestinal comfort at these higher rates of intake. Female athletes should note that the targets for carbohydrate feeding during exercise are provided in absolute amounts since it appears that the absorptive capacity of the gut is independent of body size. Thus, females may gain even greater benefits from feeding protocols during prolonged exercise than their male counterparts if the given absorption of carbohydrate can be spread across a smaller muscle mass.

Events of ~45- to 75-minute duration are not associated with limitations of muscle fuel supply when adequate preparation has been achieved. However, new research has shown that the frequent intake of small amounts of carbohydrate during exercise is associated with better performance in such protocols. It appears that there is communication between receptors in the mouth/throat and centres of reward and motor control in the brain which promote a lower perception of effort and allow higher pacing. These findings have been incorporated into new competition fuelling recommendations for athletes (Table 4.2). All feeding strategies should be well practiced during training sessions, since this may be associated with an adaptation of the gut as well as the opportunity to individualize and fine-tune the competition-fuelling plan. Of course, the practicalities of fuelling during any event are determined by event characteristics (e.g., access to feed zones or aid stations, rules that provide breaks in play, opportunities to transport own supplies).

The other major nutritional strategy during exercise involves replacement of the fluid lost in sweat. Sweat losses vary during exercise according to such factors as the duration and intensity of exercise, environmental conditions, and the acclimatization of the athlete, but typically range between 500 and 2000 mL/h. As the resulting fluid deficit increases, however, it gradually increases the stress associated with exercise, such as the drifting increase in heart rate and perception of effort. The point at which this causes a noticeable or significant impairment of exercise capacity and performance will depend on the individual, the environment (effects are greater in the heat or at altitude), and the type of exercise. The general recommendations are that an athlete use the opportunities that are specific to her sport to replace as much of her sweat loss as is practical during the event, with the general goal of keeping the fluid deficit below 2% of body mass in stressful environments. Checking body mass before and after the session and then accounting for the weight of drinks and foods consumed during the session will allow the athlete to calculate her sweat rates, rates of fluid replacement, and the total sweat deficit over the session. This can be useful in developing and fine-tuning an individualized hydration plan that is specific to an event and its conditions.

Since studies find that athletes typically replace only 30–60% of fluid losses across a range of sporting activities, many athletes may find an improvement in performance with a competition nutrition plan that better integrates their fluid and carbohydrate goals across their event. However, recent observations from sporting events attracting large numbers of recreational participants have shown that there is a need specifically to warn against drinking excessively before and during exercise. Slower participants in running, cycling, and triathlon races have been observed to consume fluids at rates that greatly exceed their sweat losses—combining low sweat rates with aggressive use of aid stations during the event. Such drinking patterns, which can lead to a weight gain over the race, are a major risk factor for the development of hyponatremia (low plasma sodium concentrations). Several athletes have died in marathons as a result of severe hyponatremia. Females appear to be at greater risk of over-drinking during exercise than male athletes—perhaps as a result of their smaller size/lower sweat rates and their greater effort to follow what they think are healthy/beneficial patterns. Assessing actual sweat rates and fluid intakes during training sessions will help to ensure than an appropriate competition plan is developed.

Recovery between competitive events

Many sporting competitions require the athlete to perform more than once to decide the eventual outcome. These scenarios include cycling stage races and tournaments in team or racket sports, as well as the heats and finals in many shorter events such as swimming, rowing, and track and field competition. Depending on the event, the athlete may need to recover from fluid losses, fuel depletion, muscle damage, and other challenges to performance. Being able to recover well—or at least better than her opponent—will be a key issue in performing well at the most important time.

The main dietary factor in postevent refueling is the amount of carbohydrate consumed. Since glycogen storage may occur at a slightly faster rate during the first couple of hours after exercise, athletes are often advised to begin refueling immediately after exercise. However, the main reason for promoting carbohydrate-rich meals or snacks soon after exercise is that effective refueling does not start until a substantial amount of carbohydrate (about 1 g/kg BM) is consumed (see Table 4.2). Rapid refueling strategies are important when there is less than 8 hours between exercise sessions but when recovery time is longer, immediate intake of carbohydrate after exercise is unnecessary and the athletes should choose their preferred meal/snack schedule for achieving total carbohydrate intake goals. The co-ingestion of protein with carbohydrate-rich recovery meals and snacks may enhance glycogen synthesis when the total intake of carbohydrate is below optimal targets. Nevertheless, the main reason to consume high-quality protein after exercise is to promote protein synthesis during the recovery phase. This may help to reduce muscle soreness as well as function.

Rehydration is another issue in postevent recovery since athletes can expect to be at least mildly dehydrated at the end of their session. In essence, the success of postexercise rehydration is dependent on how much the athlete drinks and then how much of this is retained and re-equilibrated within body fluid compartments. It may take 6–24 hours for complete rehydration following fluid losses of 2–5% of BM. When it is important to encourage voluntary fluid intake, flavored drinks have been shown to encourage greater intake than plain water. Urine losses appear to be minimized by the simultaneous replacement of lost electrolytes, particularly sodium. The inclusion of sodium in a rehydration drink is an important

strategy in the rapid recovery of moderate to high fluid deficits. However, the optimal sodium level is about 50–80 mmol/L, as found in oral rehydration solutions used in the treatment of diarrhea. This is considerably higher than the concentrations found in commercial sports drinks and may be unpalatable to many athletes. Alternatively, sodium can be consumed in recovery meals in the form of sodium-rich foods (e.g., bread, cheese, breakfast cereals) or by adding salt to cooking or food preparation. Creatively planned meals and snacks may be able to simultaneously provide the athlete's needs for carbohydrate, protein, fluid, and electrolytes.

Supplements and sports foods

The sports world is full of supplements and sports foods that claim to make the athlete faster, stronger, leaner, better recovered, healthier, with greater endurance, or whatever other factors are important to performance. Sports supplements include products that address the special nutritional needs of athletes. This category includes sports drinks, sports bars, liquid meal supplements, and micronutrient supplements that are part of a prescribed dietary plan. Many of these products are specially designed to help an athlete meet specific needs for energy and nutrients, including fluid and carbohydrates, in situations where everyday foods are not practical to eat. This is particularly relevant for intake immediately before, during, or after exercise. These supplements can be shown to improve performance when they allow the athlete to achieve their sports nutrition goals. However, they are more expensive than normal food, a consideration that must be balanced against the convenience they provide.

Nutritional ergogenic aids—products that promise a direct performance-enhancing effect—are the supplements that seem most appealing to athletes. In general, these supplements have been poorly tested, or have failed to live up to their claims when rigorous testing has been undertaken. Exceptions to this are creatine, caffeine, beetroot juice (nitrate supplement), and the buffering agents bicarbonate and beta-alanine. Each of these products may enhance the performance of certain athletes under specific conditions. Athletes should seek expert's advice about such supplements to see whether their sport/exercise warrants experimentation with these products and to ensure that a correct protocol is tried. The Sports Supplement Program of the Australian Institute of Sport provides information about many products, and rates supplements and sports foods into four categories based on the amount of scientific support for the claims made about the use of the product, and whether it is considered a banned substance (see http://www.ausport.gov.au/ais/nutrition). It is important to recognize that even in the case of products with good evidence of benefits, athletes should only consider supplement use after they have put in place a well-chosen eating plan.

One risk that should be considered in contemplating the use of supplements is the potential for a product to contain impurities and contaminants. Since the mid-1990s, it has become apparent that some supplements contain pro-hormones and stimulants that are banned under the World Anti-Doping Codes. While these products should be declared as ingredients on supplement labels, there is evidence that this does not occur in a substantial number of cases. In fact, the watershed study by an International Olympic Committee-accredited laboratory found that 15% of supplements contained detectable levels of banned pro-hormones that were undeclared. Situations of "contamination" can include products containing therapeutic doses of banned stimulants or steroids that are not identified on the ingredients list, presumably in order to ensure that the supplement "works." Unfortunately, these can lead to health problems—often of a serious nature. Mostly, however, the contamination occurs in trace amounts. Unfortunately, these impurities may be sufficient to cause an inadvertent doping outcome in drug testing; since the athlete faces a code of strict liability under anti-doping laws, they will be held responsible for any failed drug test even when it can be proved that they unwittingly ingested a supplement containing banned ingredients.

Special cultural issues for sports nutrition for females

The final section of this chapter will briefly consider the characteristics of foods and food combinations that may be of particular value in constructing meal plans for female athletes. This is not based on scientific evidence that particular foods provide a physiological advantage to female athletes in comparison with males. Instead, it is based on the author's experience that particular eating styles can be useful in helping female athletes meet their overall nutrient needs and nutritional goals while addressing their exercise-based carbohydrate targets. In addition, some ideas based on considerations of common food preferences of females and their relationship with food are presented.

Themes and practices that have been observed in working with female athletes are summarized in Table 4.3 and are based on two different issues. The first issue is focused on the weight management concerns and lower energy intakes of female athletes. Here, it is useful for food choices or eating practices to be characterized as low to moderate in total energy value and energy density (energy value per 100 g of food), high in protein and key micronutrients (to allow other nutritional goals to be met simultaneously), and satiating (to prevent hunger or to reduce risks of overeating). A variety of food or food combinations can address these goals (see Table 4.3 for examples). The second issue concerns common food preferences that the author has noted among female athletes which often revolve around the preference for specific foods and the inclusion of special foods or social eating occasions in dietary practices. These examples can, at best, be described as anecdotal, and it is suggested that research be undertaken to better understand the importance of culture, sex, and dietary restraint in determining the food choices of female athletes. However, it is the experience of this author that when possible, female athletes should be assisted to find foods and eating strategies that maximize whole foods, eating enjoyment and shared dining.

Summary

Female athletes have been under-represented in sports nutrition studies. Nevertheless, the available evidence suggests that the present guidelines for nutritional strategies to promote training outcomes and competition performance are suitable for female athletes. The issue of low energy availability among female athletes is not only a concern in terms of poor health and performance outcomes, but can change requirements for some nutrients. Further research should be undertaken both to confirm whether females have special sports nutrition requirements and to utilize food choices and eating strategies that are of cultural importance to females in intervention studies.

Recommended reading

Beals KA (ed). (2013) *Nutritional Needs of Female Athletes: From Research to Practice*. CRC Press, Boca Raton, FL.

Burke L. (2007) *Practical Sports Nutrition*. Human Kinetics, Champaign, IL.

Burke LM, and Deakin V (eds). (2010) *Clinical Sports Nutrition*, (4th edn). McGraw-Hill, Sydney.

Maughan RJ (eds). (2013) *The Encyclopaedia of Sports Medicine: An IOC Medical Commission Publication, Sports Nutrition*. John Wiley & Sons, London.

Chapter 5
Disordered eating and eating disorders in female athletes

Monica K. Torstveit[1] and Jorunn Sundgot-Borgen[2]

[1]Faculty of Health and Sport Sciences, University of Agder, Kristiansand, Norway
[2]The Sports Medicine Department, The Norwegian School of Sport Sciences, Oslo, Norway

Introduction

For female athletes, the desire to excel in sports has led to various methods of training, conditioning, and dietary alterations in an attempt to improve their performance. In many sports, body weight and body composition are crucial performance variables. Some female athletes are genetically suited to the specific anthropometric demands of the sport in which they compete, but many female athletes struggle with disordered eating (DE) and eating disorders (EDs) as they attempt to conform to demands or competition regulations that are ill-suited to their physique. In this situation, participation in sports may lead to an array of health concerns that may adversely affect the female athlete's short- and long-term health at a variety of performance levels and sports.

Therefore in this chapter, we will define the DE spectrum and describe the prevalence of DE and EDs among female athletes. Thereafter, risk factors and health- and performance-related consequences of DE and EDs will be presented. Finally, we discuss identification, diagnosis, and possible treatment initiatives of DE and EDs among athletes, including special considerations for the sports physician and allied health personnel.

The Female Athlete, First Edition. Edited by Margo L. Mountjoy.
© 2015 International Olympic Committee. Published 2015 by John Wiley & Sons, Inc.

Definitions

The DE continuum starts with appropriate eating and exercise behaviors, including healthy dieting (such as lowering energy intake and gradual weight loss) and the occasional use of more extreme weight loss methods such as short-term restrictive diets (<30 kcal per kg fat-free mass (FFM) per day). These behaviors may progress to chronic dieting, binging, and use of fasting, passive or active dehydration, laxatives, diuretics, vomiting, and excessive training. The continuum ends with clinical EDs, where athletes are struggling with extreme dieting, abnormal eating behavior, distorted body image, weight fluctuations, and variable athletic performance.

Athletes can be underweight, normal weight, or overweight, irrespective of the presence of DE or EDs. The purpose of DE behavior is usually to achieve a low body weight or perceived "ideal body composition" to compensate for strong body dissatisfaction. Athletes with DE often continuously feel too fat for their sport, and the DE behaviors may become more intensified, to a degree where the athlete meets the criteria for a clinical ED. The DSM-IV diagnostic criteria have recently been revised (DSM-V) and the clinical EDs include anorexia nervosa, bulimia nervosa, binge eating disorder and other specified and unspecified feeding or eating disorder (OSFED). These EDs have many features in common, and patients/athletes frequently move between them. The criteria for these disorders are listed in Tables 5.1–5.4, and a

Table 5.1 Data from DSM-V diagnostic criteria for anorexia nervosa

Diagnostic criteria for anorexia nervosa

A. Restriction of energy intake relative to requirements leading to a significantly low body weight in the context of age, sex, developmental trajectory, and physical health
B. Intense fear of gaining weight or becoming fat, even though underweight
C. Disturbance in the way in which one's body weight or shape is experienced, undue influence of body weight or shape on self-evaluation, or denial of the seriousness of the current low body weight

Table 5.2 Data from DSM-V diagnostic criteria for bulimia nervosa

Diagnostic criteria for bulimia nervosa

A. Recurrent episodes of binge eating characterized by both of the following:
    1. Eating in a discrete amount of time (within a 2-hour period) large amounts of food
    2. Sense of lack of control over eating during an episode
B. Recurrent inappropriate compensatory behavior in order to prevent weight gain (purging)
C. The binge eating and compensatory behaviors both occur, on average, at least once a week for 3 months
D. Self-evaluation is unduly influenced by body shape and weight
E. The disturbance does not occur exclusively during episodes of anorexia nervosa

Table 5.3 Data from DSM-V diagnostic criteria for binge eating disorder

Diagnostic criteria for binge eating disorder

A. Recurrent episodes of binge eating. An episode of binge eating is characterized by both of the following:
    1. Eating, in a discrete period of time (e.g., within any 2-hour period), an amount of food that is definitely larger than most people would eat in a similar period of time under similar circumstances
    2. A sense of lack of control over eating during the episode (e.g., a feeling that one cannot stop eating or control what or how much one is eating)
B. The binge eating episodes are associated with three (or more) of the following:
    1. Eating much more rapidly than normal
    2. Eating until feeling uncomfortably full
    3. Eating large amounts of food when not feeling physically hungry
    4. Eating alone because of feeling embarrassed by how much one is eating
    5. Feeling disgusted with oneself, depressed, or very guilty afterward
C. Marked distress regarding binge eating is present
D. The binge eating occurs, on average, at least once a week for 3 months
E. The binge eating is not associated with the recurrent use of inappropriate compensatory behavior (e.g., purging) and does not occur exclusively during the course anorexia nervosa, bulimia nervosa, or avoidant/restrictive food intake disorder

Table 5.4 Examples of presentations that can be specified using the "other specified" designation for the DSM-V OSFED

Diagnostic criteria for OSFED—examples

1. *Atypical anorexia nervosa*: All of the criteria for anorexia nervosa are met, except that despite significant weight loss, the individual's weight is within or above the normal range
2. *Bulimia nervosa (of low frequency and/or limited duration):* All of the criteria for bulimia nervosa are met, except that the binge eating and inappropriate compensatory behaviors occur, on average, less than once a week and/or for less than 3 months.
3. *Binge eating disorder (of low frequency and/or limited duration):* All of the criteria for binge eating disorder are met, except the binge eating occurs, on average, less than once a week and/or for less than 3 months.
4. *Purging disorder:* Recurrent purging behavior to influence weight or shape (e.g., self-induced vomiting, misuse of laxatives, diuretics, or other medications) in the absence of binge eating
5. *Night eating syndrome:* Recurrent episodes of night eating, as manifested by eating after awakening from sleep or by excessive food consumption after the evening meal. There is awareness and recall of the eating. The night eating is not better explained by external influences such as changes in the individual's sleep–wake cycle or by local social norms. The night eating causes significant distress and/or impairment in functioning. The disordered pattern of eating is not better explained by binge eating disorder or another mental disorder, including substance use, and is not attributable to another medical disorder or to an effect of medication

short description of the disorders and the changes in the new DSM-V criteria follows below.

Anorexia nervosa primarily affects adolescent girls and young women and is characterized by distorted body image with a pathological fear of becoming fat that leads to excessive dieting and severe weight loss. The DSM-V criteria have several minor but important changes from the DSM-IV criteria. Criterion A focuses on behavior like restricting calorie intake and no longer includes the word "refusal" in terms of weight maintenance, since that implies intention on the part of the patient and can be difficult to assess. The DSM-IV Criterion D requiring amenorrhea or the absence of at least three menstrual cycles, as well as the weight criterion, has been deleted.

Bulimia nervosa is characterized by frequent episodes of binge eating followed by behaviors such as self-induced vomiting, abuse of laxatives, diuretics or other medications, fasting, or excessive exercise to avoid weight gain. The number of binge episodes to meet the diagnostic criteria for bulimia nervosa has been reduced to one time per week in the DSM-V version.

Binge eating disorder is defined as recurring episodes of eating significantly more food in a short period of time than most people would eat under similar circumstances, with episodes marked by feelings of lack of control. The person may have feelings of guilt, embarrassment, or disgust, and may binge eat alone to hide the behavior. This disorder is associated with marked distress and occurs, on average, at least once a week over three months. This change from the DSM-IV is intended to increase awareness of the substantial differences between binge eating disorder and the common phenomenon of overeating. While overeating is a challenge for many, recurrent binge eating is much less common, far more severe and is associated with significant physical and psychological problems.

OSFED acknowledges the existence and importance of a variety of eating disturbances and is characterized as disturbances in eating behavior that do not necessarily fall into the specific category of anorexia nervosa, bulimia nervosa, or binge eating disorder. OSFED can cause clinically significant distress or impairment in social, occupational, or other important areas of functioning.

Implication of the new DSM-V criteria

The goal of reducing the number of EDNOS cases was accomplished in the DSM-V by adding new categories such as OSFED and binge eating disorder, and by changing the criteria for anorexia nervosa and bulimia nervosa. While these changes make it easier to meet the criteria for an ED, it also helps athletes get the care they need at an earlier stage to improve both treatment and prognosis. It is essential for athletes experiencing DE or EDs to have a diagnosis that accurately describes their symptoms and behaviors, since determining an accurate diagnosis is the first step for clinicians and patients in defining a treatment plan for the eating disordered "injured" athlete.

Prevalence

Although a number of studies have reported suboptimal energy and nutrient intake in weight-sensitive sports, the prevalence of athletes with low energy availability (LEA) without DE or EDs has not been evaluated. This is due to the lack of standardization related to the assessment of LEA. In terms of DE, a recent review including female athletes (not only elite athletes) and non-athletes aged between 12 and 35 years concluded that most studies (12 of 22 studies) showed no significant difference between the athlete group and the control group regarding the presence of DE. These results were based on studies done in 11 countries and most studies used self-reporting questionnaires to screen for DE. Furthermore, among the five studies that extended the methods from using only questionnaires to adding a clinical interview to diagnose EDs, three found a higher prevalence in the athlete group than in the control group.

A controlled study using clinical interview to diagnose EDs (DSM-IV) found a higher prevalence rate of EDs among Norwegian female elite athletes in leanness sports (47%) than among athletes in nonleanness sports (20%) and among nonathletic controls (21%). The prevalence of EDs (DSM-IV) among female adolescent elite athletes and controls has been estimated to 13.5% versus 5.1%, respectively, indicating a lower prevalence than in the adult elite athletes. In aesthetic sports (e.g., gymnastics, ballet, and figure skating), the prevalence of EDs is estimated to be about 40%, and in weight-class sports about 30% for elite female athletes. In contrast, the prevalence in team sports is about 15% in elite female athletes, while corresponding values in technical sports are about 17%.

It is important to remember that methodological considerations should be emphasized when discussing the prevalence of DE and EDs among athletes. Nevertheless, in studies using clinical evaluation, the prevalence of EDs among female athletes is much higher than that reported in self-report studies, and DE and EDs appear to be more frequent among adult female athletes competing in sports focusing on leanness and/or a low weight than among athletes competing in sports where these factors are considered less important.

Risk factors

Of the few studies reporting on risk factors for developing EDs in athletes, most show that elite athletes have a greater risk of developing EDs than nonelite athletes and controls. However, the reason why some athletes cross the line from dieting to clinical EDs is not yet known. It is generally accepted that the pathogenesis of EDs is multifactorial with cultural, individual, familial, and genetic/biochemical factors playing roles. In addition, there are factors specific to the athletic community, such as dieting to enhance performance, personality factors (such as perfectionism, obsessiveness), pressure to lose weight, frequent weight cycling, early start of sport-specific training, overtraining, recurrent and non-healing injuries, unfortunate coaching behavior, and regulations in some sports.

In aesthetic sports, comments made by coaches on an athlete's body can be associated with a psychological pressure to start dieting, and there is a common belief that judges are influenced by the body composition or shape of the athlete. Although social pressure is the strongest predictor

of DE in nonelite athletes and controls, in elite athletes, the strongest predictor seems to be body image dissatisfaction. Recently, it has been reported that athletes who were dissatisfied with their body and athletes who reported dieting and the desire to be leaner to improve performance were more likely to develop EDs than athletes who were less dissatisfied with their body. Furthermore, parental influences, rather than self-esteem, are predictors of DE in elite athletes, unlike for nonelite athletes and nonathletes.

Injured athletes often experience undesired weight gain, combined with the negative effects that injuries may cause (e.g., not being able to train and compete), leading to increased risk for EDs. Furthermore, it is suggested that pressures on athletes to reduce weight and body fat can lead to a culture of DE. The result is that in some of the weight-sensitive sports, there might be an indirect increased risk for EDs. It is important to have in mind that to examine the true risk and triggers of participation in sports on the development of EDs, controlled, longitudinal studies are needed. In order to identify the at-risk athletes as early as possible, knowledge of signs and symptoms is necessary, and for that reason, an overview of physical/medical and psychological/behavioral characteristics of DE/EDs among athletes is presented in Table 5.5.

Health and performance consequences

Health consequences

Every organ system can be affected by an ED, but to our knowledge, there are no studies that have specifically examined the short- and long-term health consequences of DE or EDs in athletes. However, it is reasonable to expect that the health consequences reported among nonathletes will also apply to athletes.

Clinical EDs may cause serious medical problems that in some circumstances can be fatal. Health complications of DE and EDs involve the cardiovascular, gastrointestinal, endocrine, reproductive, skeletal, renal, and central nervous systems,

Table 5.5 Physical/medical symptoms and psychological/behavioral characteristics of DE/EDs among female athletes

Physical/medical	Characteristics
Dermatological/dental	Hair loss
	Dry skin, brittle hair and nails
	Lanugo hair
	Dorsal hand callus or abrasions
	Dental and gum problems
Cardiovascular	Bradycardia
	Hypotension
Endocrine	Hypoglycemia
	Delayed onset of puberty
	Menstrual dysfunction
	Reduced bone mass/stress fractures
Gastrointestinal	Swollen parotid glands
	Constipation, diarrhea, bloating
	Postprandial distress
Renal	Dehydration
	Edema
	Electrolyte disturbances
	Hypokalemia
	Muscle cramps
	Metabolic alkalosis
Other	Significant weight loss/frequent weight fluctuations
	Fatigue
	Anemic
	Hypothermia
Psychological/ behavioral	
	Restrictive eating, binging, and purging
	Avoidance of eating/eating situation
	Dissatisfaction with body image (especially in the sport context)/self-critical (especially concerning body, weight, and sport performance)
	Low self-esteem
	Poor coping skills
	Mood swings
	Extreme performance orientation
	Perfectionistic
	Compulsive and excessive training, also when injured and Restlessness; relaxing is difficult or impossible
	Insomnia
	Reduced social activities
	Poor concentration
	Resistance to weight gain or maintenance recommended by sport support staff
	Anxiety
	Depression

including psychological stress and depressions (see Table 5.6). Most complications of anorexia nervosa, such as depletion of muscle glycogen stores, loss of muscle mass and bone mass, and anemia, occur as a direct or indirect result of starvation.

Osteopenia and osteoporosis are among the most severe and common complications of prolonged LEA and anorexia nervosa. These conditions are associated with fragility fractures and stress fractures, even in the young population. Severe complications such as collapse of the femoral head and hip fracture have been reported even among athletes.

The consequences of bulimia nervosa have not been studied as extensively as anorexia nervosa, possibly due to more normal ranging body weight values and because it is a more difficult problem to diagnose. While multiple neuroendocrine abnormalities may be present, they tend to be less pronounced than with anorexia nervosa. Complications of bulimia nervosa relate mainly to binge eating and purging. The loss of fluids and electrolytes during purging can result in serious medical problems such as acid-base abnormalities, cardiac rhythm disturbances, and dehydration. The variety of medical problems related to bulimia nervosa includes tooth decay, parotid enlargement, carpopedal spasm, stomach rupture, metabolic alkalosis, hypercarotenemia, hypokalemia, and pancreatitis. Menstrual dysfunction and impaired bone health are also present in this group, but the incidence is highly variable and seems to increase with the presence of previous anorexia nervosa. The weight gain related to binge eating will likely lead to the same medical problems in athletes as in nonathletes, especially in those athletes participating in the more technical, less endurance type sports. Furthermore, the risk of overuse injuries and other muscle skeletal problems is likely higher than in nonbinging athletes.

In the sports medicine field, the relationship between energy availability, menstrual function, and bone health is referred to as the female athlete triad (the Triad). Each clinical condition of the Triad comprises the pathologic end of a spectrum of interrelated subclinical conditions between health and disease (e.g., a spectrum of energy availability from optimal energy availability to

Table 5.6 A presentation of possible health- and performance-related consequences associated with various extreme weight control behaviors and DE/EDs

Weight control behavior	Physiological effects and health consequences	Effect on performance
Fasting or starvation	Energy and nutrient deficiency, glycogen depletion, loss of lean body mass, decreased metabolic rate, and reduced BMD.	Poor exercise performance due to general weakness, reduced ability to cope with pressure, decreased muscle force, and increased susceptibility for diseases and injuries.
Diet pills	Typically function by suppressing appetite and may cause a slight increase in metabolic rate. May induce rapid heart rate, anxiety, nervousness, inability to sleep, and dehydration. Any weight lost is quickly regained once use is discontinued.	May indirectly result in poor performance and may be classified as doping.
Laxatives or enemas	Weight loss is primarily water and any weight lost is regained once use is discontinued. Dehydration and electrolyte imbalances, constipation, cathartic colon, and steatorrhea are common.	May affect concentration and hydration status. May be addictive and the athlete can develop resistance, thus requiring larger and larger doses to produce the same effect.
Diuretics	Weight loss is primarily water and any weight lost is quickly regained once use is discontinued. Dehydration and electrolyte imbalances are not uncommon.	Poor exercise performance and classified as doping.
Self-induced vomiting	Large body water losses can lead to dehydration and electrolyte imbalances. Gastrointestinal problems, including esophagitis, esophageal perforation, and esophageal ulcers may occur.	Poor exercise performance. Largely ineffective in promoting weight (body fat) loss.
Saunas	Dehydration and electrolyte imbalances can occur in extreme cases.	Weight loss is primarily water and any weight lost is quickly regained once fluids are replaced.
Excessive exercise	If combined with LEA, it will increase the risk of staleness, chronic fatigue, illness, overuse, injury, and menstrual dysfunction.	May experience the effect of lack of recovery.

LEA with or without an ED). Although any one of these problems can occur in isolation, the emphasis on weight loss and/or LEA in individuals at risk can start a cycle in which all three problems occur in sequence. In recent years, studies have found the Triad in elite athletes representing both leanness and nonleanness sports, in female college athletes and high-school athletes, as well as in women who are not competing in sports. A study of the entire population of female elite athletes in Norway demonstrated that 4.3% of female elite athletes met all the criteria for the Triad. When evaluating the presence of two of the components of the Triad, prevalence ranged from 5% to as high as 27% in elite athletes, indicating that the consequences of LEA is widespread among female athletes. Therefore, we recommend that health personnel working with female athletes look closely for evidence of Triad disorders.

It should also be noted that an additional component of Triad disorders, endothelial dysfunction, has recently been introduced in the literature. Endothelial dysfunction is an important factor in the pathogenesis of cardiovascular disease, which needs further examination in future studies on athletes.

In terms of mortality rates, a meta-analysis found an elevated mortality rate for patients with all types of EDs (DSM-IV). The highest risk of death was found in patients with anorexia nervosa, who had a weighted annual mortality rate of 5 per 1000 persons per years, followed by patients with EDNOS (3 per 1000 persons per years), and patients with bulimia nervosa (1.7 per 1000 persons per years). A number of deaths related to EDs among top-level athletes representing gymnastics, running, alpine skiing, and cycling have been reported in the media, but mortality rates of EDs among athletes have not been published. However, among Norwegian female elite athletes, 5.4% ($n = 5$) of those diagnosed with EDs reported suicide attempts.

Implications for the young athlete

Due to the biological changes occurring during adolescence, it is important to remember that the body of a young growing athlete often develops in a direction counter to the demands of the athlete's sport. This is especially true in females and particularly in sports where leanness or a low body weight is considered important for optimal performance. The development of EDs typically begins at the age of about 14–17 years when athletes specialize in a particular sport. Long-term LEA and insufficient nutrient intakes during the growth period can lead to delayed pubertal development and retarded growth. Delayed menarche, bone growth retardation, reduced height, weight, and body fat have been reported in gymnasts. The consequences of long-term LEA are particularly severe for the adolescent athlete, since the imbalance of bone remodeling prevents optimal peak bone mass, stature, and development of the reproductive system.

Performance consequences

It goes without saying that health should be more important than performance for the athlete and their respective team. Unfortunately, our experience working with elite athletes with EDs has shown us that the athletes often see it the opposite way. For them, a focus on performance-related consequences may provide more incentive to improve than a focus on the health consequences in terms of being willing to cooperate in a treatment program. Therefore, we believe it is very important for health personnel to have knowledge of performance-related consequences of EDs and use this knowledge when approaching and helping the female athletes with DE or EDs. The effect of DE or EDs on athletic performance depends on several factors

such as the severity of the DE practices, the age of the athlete, the type, duration, and severity of the ED, as well as the type of sport or event that the athlete participates in.

It has been shown that cortisol maintains plasma glucose concentration by breaking down skeletal muscle into amino acids for gluconeogenesis in the liver. Stimuli such as starvation or intense training leading to reduced plasma glucose concentration may therefore result in atrophy, leading to decreased muscle strength and power and an increased injury risk. Endurance performance is likely to be impaired if the liver and muscle glycogen levels are lower or if the athlete is dehydrated or anemic. Further, acute dehydration can lead to loss of motor skills and coordination, while a reduced blood volume may impair thermoregulatory capacity during exercise, which can lead to impaired performance. A Norwegian study reported negative consequences from 2 months of LEA on cardiovascular function and performance, showing that maximum oxygen uptake and running speed of elite female endurance athletes were decreased for several months.

If purging methods place the athlete in a state of LEA and psychological stress, then the potential effects on performance are similar to those seen with chronic or severe energy restriction. In addition to causing energy and nutrient deficiencies, purging poses some unique problems regarding athletic performance, including most notably dehydration and severe electrolyte imbalances. Electrolyte imbalances may slow nerve conduction velocity and muscle contraction leading to increased reaction times and reduced recovery rates. Electrolyte abnormalities over time may also lead to a loss of muscle mass followed by decreased strength and power. Other consequences related to fluid and electrolyte imbalances not coincident with peak performance are fatigue, light-headedness, insomnia, and reduced ability to concentrate (Table 5.6).

Low self-esteem, depression, and anxiety disorders are psychological problems associated with EDs. For athletes, the stress of constantly obsessing about food, denying hunger, agonizing over body weight, and fearing increased body weight can be mentally exhausting. It is clear that this preoccupation can interfere with the athlete's daily activities as well as athletic performance.

Special considerations

One challenge for health personnel, coaches, and athletes is that some who severely restrict their energy intake for short periods and lose weight do experience an initial, albeit transient, improvement in performance. One explanation may be due to the initial physiological and psychological consequences of starvation where the athlete may feel lighter due to weight loss and thus experience a psychological boost, particularly when competing in sports in which being lighter can correlate with improved performance. Possible health- and performance-related consequences to various extreme weight control behaviors and/or DE/EDs in athletes are listed in Table 5.6.

Identification, diagnosis, and treatment

Managing the athlete with an ED is challenging from a medical, psychological, and sport environment standpoint. Most athletes will only divulge their symptoms when asked directly by their coach, teammates, or sport physician and allied health personnel. Some will even deny claims about possible DE or ED behaviors. Therefore, professionals working with athletes should have knowledge about possible risk factors and early signs and symptoms of DE/EDs (Table 5.5), along with the health- and performance-related consequences of DE/EDs (Table 5.6), and how to approach the problem if it occurs (Tables 5.7–5.10).

Identification

Early detection of DE and EDs is important because like most conditions, EDs become harder to treat as they progress. However, early detection of these conditions among athletes is often difficult since self-reporting of DE and EDs is rare, possibly due to secrecy, shame, denial, and fear of reprisal. Several standardized, self-report screening questionnaires especially designed to screen for DE and/or EDs exist. The most well-known are the Eating Disorder Inventory, the Eating Disorder Examination Questionnaire, the Eating Attitudes Test, and the SCOFF questionnaire. These instruments have been validated in the general population, but are not well enough tested for sensitivity or validity with athletes. Hence, the resultant information may not be accurate in the athletic population. Even though self-report questionnaires are valuable and easy to use, it is recommended that they are complemented with other information-gathering tools, such as in-depth personal interviews.

Based on our experience working with adolescent elite and national team athletes with DE or suspected EDs talking to them about menstruation, training, or injuries is less threatening for them than questions regarding body weight, dieting or food and has often revealed the presence of DE. A dialogue to initiate discussion might include some of the eight questions included in the International Olympic Committee (IOC)-endorsed Periodic Health Examination developed to screen for the Triad:
- Have you ever had a menstrual period?
- What was your age at your first menstrual period?
- Do you have regular menstrual periods?
- How many menstrual cycles did you have in the last year?
- When was your most recent menstrual period?
- Have you had a stress fracture in the past?
- Have you ever been identified as having a problem with low bone density (osteopenia or osteoporosis)?
- Are you presently taking any female hormones (estrogen, progesterone, birth control pills)?

Furthermore, we also recommend questions presented in Table 5.7 being considered in the conversation with the athletes.

Special considerations

Even though most research has concluded that EDs are more prevalent among female athletes representing leanness sport compared with non-leanness sports, EDs are also a challenge to athletes representing sports that do not focus on thinness and

Table 5.7 Questions that can be included in the consultation

Questions about food	Questions about weight	Questions about menstruation	Questions about training and injuries
Do you feel that you have a "relaxed" relation to food?	What have your highest and lowest body weight been during the last year?	When did you experience your first menstruation?	Please describe your normal training volume (frequency, intensity, duration)
Please describe your eating habits[1]	What would you say your "competition" body weight is?	Have your periods been regular since you first began menstruating?	Have you altered training methods, volume, or intensity recently (or in the past)?
How many meals do you eat per day?	Have you lost weight recently? How did you achieve the weight loss?	What is the longest period of time you have experienced lack of menstrual bleeding?	Do you practice any exercise in addition to your sport-specific training?
Are there any types of food you try to avoid or do you have any "forbidden" foods?	Are you comfortable with your current body weight?	When was your last period?	Have you had any problems with overuse injuries? What type of injuries?
Can you tell me what you ate and drank yesterday?	Are there other people who are especially interested in your body weight?	How do you feel about having/ not having menstruation?[2]	Have you ever had a stress fracture or a normal fracture?
Possibly question the athlete about purging methods (preferably referring to the past)		Do you currently use oral contraceptive pills or other contraceptives? Have you used them in the past?	When experiencing an injury, did you take time to recover? How did you feel about that?

[1]It can be difficult for one with eating problems to spontaneously list what she has eaten. An athlete with anorexia nervosa avoids fat and is often a vegetarian. Eating habits are characterized by the same restrictive intake of "acceptable" foods each day. A person with bulimia nervosa constantly attempts to postpone calorie consumption then overeats in the afternoon and evening.

[2]An athlete with an ED prefers not to menstruate (many feel it is a "defeat" to have, in their belief, such high-percent body fat that one has regular menstruation).

a low body weight. Athletes competing in sports such as ball game (e.g., soccer, volleyball, and team handball) and power sports (e.g., alpine skiing, weight lifting, and shot put) are also affected by DE and EDs, but more often related to bulimic behaviors, rather than anorexia nervosa. It is extremely important to note that thinness is not an essential sign of an ED. In fact, most athletes struggling with EDs are normal weight, some are underweight, and some are even overweight. However, most athletes on the DE spectrum look "normal" in terms of body weight and shape.

Another important consideration is the age of the athlete. Most studies have investigated adult athletes, but recent studies have shown a higher prevalence of EDs among adolescent elite athletes compared with age-matched nonathletic controls. Therefore, focus should also be placed on younger athletes (high school age) in terms of screening and identification of these problems. Finally, an important question is when to screen for DE and EDs. Prime opportunities include the pre-participation exam, an annual checkup, or any time an athlete is evaluated for a related problem, such as recurrent injury, stress fracture, amenorrhea, or illness. Symptoms to look for are presented under the "Diagnosis" section, in Table 5.8.

Diagnosis

Following screening, accurate diagnosis of EDs is dependent on a thorough evaluation of the athlete by the physician and other members of an experienced multidisciplinary healthcare team.

Physical examination signs such as low BMI/ low percentage of body fat, bradycardia, lanugo, hypercarotenemia, or other signs of an ED should prompt further evaluation. In Table 5.8,

Table 5.8 The anthropometric, biochemical, clinical, dietary, and environmental (ABCDE) assessment of athletes with DE/EDs by healthcare professionals

ABCDEs	Measures	Comments
Anthropometric	Body height Body mass Body composition Girth and breadths	Valid and reliable methods of body composition should be sought (e.g., DXA, skinfold assessment using the International Society for Kinanthropometry (ISAK) standards; four component models assessing fat, fat free, and lean tissue mass, and total body water; measurement of hydration status recommended for all anthropometric assessments). Careful reflection required whether assessment of body mass and composition may trigger more problems.
Biochemical	Complete blood count Complete metabolic panel Lipid panel Iron profile Thyroid function (e.g., TSH and T3) Estradiol, progesterone, prolactin, LH, and FSH Cortisol 25 (OH) vitamin D Urine analysis Pregnancy test	In females with menstrual dysfunction, prolactin needs to be assessed to rule out pituitary tumor; if ovarian cysts and oligomenorrhea, androgens should be assessed.
Clinical	History Physical exam Medications Dietary supplements	Medical history should include previous DE and EDs. If pre-participation physical, general medical history, including menstrual history/status, bone health, history of stress fracture and other injuries, osteoporosis. Screening for DE and EDs with screening tools or clinical interview and identification of physical signs and symptoms (e.g., general [weight fluctuations, fatigue, appetite, sleep, edema], skin [dryness, callus on hands], hair [loss, lanugo], GI symptoms [constipation, diarrhea, pain, reflux, teeth, sore mouth/tongue], cardiopulmonary [heart rate, sleep apnea, blood pressure], renal [polydipsia, color], musculoskeletal [pain, injuries, bone mass]; immune [frequent illness]; other [parotid artery enlargement]; weight fluctuations, pressure to lose weight, highest/lowest body mass at current height. Medications [oral contraceptives, antidepressants, thyroid medication]. Dietary and sport supplements [e.g., vitamins, mineral, energy-containing supplements and ergogenic aids, stimulants].
Dietary	Quantity Quality Timing Energy expenditure	Energy intake, total daily energy expenditure, resting metabolic rate, exercise energy expenditure, energy availability, energy density; macronutrients (expressed in gram/kilogram per day) and micronutrients, fluid balance, and hydration, including sweat rate, food restrictions, allergies, intolerance; scary foods; nutrient and fluid timing; carbohydrate availability during intense training; carbohydrate and fiber related to appetite; recovery nutrition; competition preparation and fueling, travel nutrition and appetite issues during travel or intense training. Dietary assessment methods: consider validity and reliability as well as additional burden and stress on DE/ED athlete when using diaries and food logs.
Environmental	Culture of sport Annual training plan and peaking Travel Work/school Family/home Experience in sport	At risk for DE/ED? Target-specific issues such as weight-making or body image depending on sport; evaluation of training/competition plan in discussion with coach; countries at risk for inadequate food access and food safety concerns; work/school schedules and time for food preparation, eating, recovery; level of athlete and experience.

an example of the anthropometric, biochemi-cal, clinical, dietary, and environmental (ABCDE) assessment is presented.

Special considerations

Unfortunately, it is often rare for an athlete to admit an eating problem during the first consul-tation. Generally, the athlete may describe symp-toms that do not necessarily point to an ED, such as headaches, constipation, diarrhea, sleeping problems, breathing problems, dizziness, sadness, or tiredness. They may complain that others make suspicious comments about their eating behavior, their weight loss, or related issues. Regardless of which complaints or symptoms are presented dur-ing the first consultation, healthcare professionals should search for underlying causes. Questions about food intake, dieting methods, and training should be straightforward and concrete. When discussing potential EDs, the athlete may feel less threatened if the discussion focuses on the past (see also Table 5.7).

Treatment

Controlled treatment studies among athletes with EDs have not been published. Therefore, our recommendations are based on the results from treatment studies on nonathletes with EDs and the authors' experience working with elite athletes.

Treatment of an athlete with EDs should utilize a multidisciplinary intervention, which normally includes a physician, a gynecologist, a nutrition-ist, a physical therapist, an exercise scientist, and in some cases, a psychiatrist or a psychologist. In addition, coaches and parents can be part of the treatment team if they have a positive rela-tionship with the athlete. The younger the ath-lete, the more the involvement of the family is recommended. The primary goals of treatment recommended by the IOC position stand on the Triad should be to optimize energy availability, to control and manage the athlete's DE behavior, to restore normal hormone levels, and to monitor

and treat other medical complications resulting from the ED.

When treating an athlete with an ED, it is important to establish that each treatment group member has a clear understanding of their responsibilities and that the group members com-municate well. As long as there are no complex underlying conflicts contributing to cause the ED, regular and long-term follow-up by a nutritionist is usually sufficient. Often though, complicating medical factors are present, and therefore, the physician should remain central in the follow-up process. The physician should be responsible for providing guidelines with respect to training during the treatment period and should consider an athlete suffering from an ED as an "injured" athlete.

In the author's experience, it is easier to estab-lish a trusting relationship when the DE/ED ath-letes believe their healthcare professional knows their sport, in addition to being trained in treat-ing these disorders. Healthcare professionals who have good knowledge about DE/EDs and know the various sports will better understand the ath-letes training setting, daily demands, and rela-tions that are specific to the sport/sport event and competitive level. Building such a relation-ship includes respecting the athlete's desire to be lean for athletic performance and express a will-ingness to work together to help the DE/ED ath-lete to become lean and healthy. The treatment team needs to accept the athlete's fears and irra-tional thoughts about food and weight and then present a rational approach for achieving self-management of healthy diet, weight, and training programs.

Among athletes, there is limited evidence related to the effect of different treatment methods. However, based on the recommendations from the IOC position stand on the Triad, we present pos-sible treatment methods in Table 5.9.

Training and competition recommendations during treatment

For athletes who agree to treatment, eligibility to continue training while symptomatic should be determined on an individual basis by treatment

Table 5.9 Possible treatment methods of athletes with DE/EDs

Types of treatment	Contents
Individual psychotherapy	The therapist works with the DE athlete and intends to: • Determine the nature of the individual's eating difficulties and how they might be most effectively changed. • Implement a change process. • Teach the athlete to deal with how her sport or sport participation may be contributing to the maintenance of the DE.
Group therapy	• The athlete is part of a group made up of other ED athletes. • Athletes discover that others have a similar problem. • Gives the individual a support group that understands her feelings and eating problem. • Provides a safe environment for the athlete to practice the new skills and attitudes she has learned.
Family therapy	• Includes the patient and her immediate family. • The family is the focus of treatment. • A goal is to modify maladaptive family interactions, attitudes, and dynamics to decrease the need for, or the function of, the DE in the family.
Nutritional counselling	• Often part of a multimodal treatment approach. • Athletes with DE do not remember what constitutes a balanced meal or "normal" eating. • The dietician's primary roles involve providing nutritional information and assisting in meal planning.
Pharmacotherapy	Can be useful in some cases, especially with patients with bulimic behaviors.

Source: Reproduced with permission from Sundgot-Borgen (2002).

staff. At minimum, the athletes should be cleared medically and psychologically, their training should not be used as a means to diet or control weight, and they should be required to follow a prescribed set of health maintenance criteria. These criteria, previously published in the IOC position stand on the Triad, have to be individual and generally include, but are not limited to, the following: (a) being in treatment, complying with the treatment plan, and progressing toward therapeutic goals, (b) maintaining a weight of at least 90% of expected, and in accordance with Behnke's theoretical concept of minimal body mass, a body fat >6% for male athletes and >12% for female athletes, or more if prescribed by the treatment team, and (c) eating enough to comply with the treatment plan regarding weight gain or weight maintenance. Sometimes negotiation with athletes is important in areas of energy intake and return to training and competition. Thus, referring to the IOC position stand, in the case of EDs, the "eligibility to continue training and competition while symptomatic would be determined on an individual basis by the treatment staff." In a recent publication, an Ad Hoc Research Working Group on Body Composition Health and Performance, under the auspices of the IOC Medical Commission also suggests declaring athletes with DE or ED as "injured." Furthermore, the group suggests a modified version of the recommendations for raising alarm and "no start" criteria that have been developed and used at the Norwegian Olympic Training Center (Table 5.10). It is recommended that support staff in other countries also follow these guidelines or use them as a starting point for further developing their management of this complex problem.

It must be emphasized that the ED treatment team makes every decision with the athletes' health as a priority. For athletes willing to follow the recommended treatment and include their coach (if athlete and coach have a good relationship) and also the parents (if appropriate) in the treatment, the compliance and prognosis is generally good. The athlete may return to competition when goal weight or body composition is reached, and they are mentally prepared and really want to compete. For athletes who refuse treatment, both training and competition should be withheld until they agree to participate.

Table 5.10 Guidelines for restricted training and competitions for athletes with DE or EDs developed by Skårderud *et al.* (2012) and used by the Norwegian Olympic Training Center

General guidelines	Specific guidelines	
	"Red light"; Always ban from competition	"Yellow light"; Sometimes ban from competition
• Health prior performance • Young athletes have stricter guidelines due to the serious health implications • Decisions are made by the team and in dialogue with the athlete and important others (e.g., family, coach) • Written agreements (contracts) • Not only the athlete, but co-athletes and team as well, are considered in these decisions	• Anorexia nervosa • Serious physical complications of the weight loss/LEA • Other serious eating disorders, for example, severe bulimia nervosa • At least three of the criteria described as "Yellow Light"	• Women: BMI below 18.5 kg/m^2 and/or body fat% below 12% and amenorrhea (below 14% for athletes under 18 years). • Men: BMI below 18.5 kg/m^2 and/or body fat% below 5% and low testosterone (below 7% for athletes under 18 years). • Amenorrhea $\geq$ 6 months (3 months for athletes under 18 years). • Reduced BMD (either from last measurement or from Z-score $\leq$ −1). • Athletes with physical complications based on the medical professional assessment, such as electrolyte imbalance or anemia. • Fatigue fracture should always be assessed as a possible expression of low energy over time. • Uncooperative athletes or those showing a lack of progress in treatment. • Athletes clearly having a negative effect on other team members by exhibiting exercise behaviors such as restrictive eating, maintenance of low weight, and excessive focus on matters pertaining to weight and food. • Athletes unable to maintain a positive energy balance over time, unresponsive to training, showing fatigue and intolerance. • Athletes participating in activities that perpetuate their eating disorder.

Summary and recommendations

Sports and physical activity is healthy for females at all ages when carried out appropriately and should be promoted for both health benefits and enjoyment. However, DE and EDs are challenges among some female athletes at different performance levels, in a variety of sports. In terms of **risk factors**, it is generally accepted that the pathogenesis of EDs is multifactorial, but the reason why some athletes cross the line from dieting to clinical EDs is not yet known. Female athletes should undergo annual screening in order to make early **identification** possible. Self-report questionnaires are useful, but not necessarily alone. We should not restrict screening to elite athletes, leanness athletes, or older athletes, and there is a value in screening younger athletes. The **diagnosis** of an ED in female athletes can easily be missed unless specifically searched for. If untreated, EDs can have long-lasting physiological and psychological **consequences** for both health and performance. **Treating** athletes with EDs should be undertaken only by qualified healthcare

professionals. Ideally, these individuals should also be familiar with and have an appreciation for the sport environment. Finally, potential treatment initiatives should be multidisciplinary in origin and be initiated as early as possible. Early identification and management is extremely important, and the future challenge is aimed mainly at the prevention of EDs among female athletes.

Reference

Sundgot-Borgen J. (2002) Disordered eating. In: ML Ireland and E Nattiv (eds), *The Female Athlete* (pp. 237–248). Saunders, Philadelphia, PA

Recommended reading

American Psychiatric Association (APA). (2013) Feeding and Eating Disorders. In *Diagnostic and Statistical Manual of Mental Disorders*, (5th edn, pp. 329–354). APA, Washington, DC.

Arcelus J, Mitchell AJ, Wales J, and Nielsen S. (2011) Mortality rates in patients with anorexia nervosa and other eating disorders: a meta-analysis of 36 studies. *Arch Gen Psychiatry*, 68(7), 724–731.

Bonci CM, Bonci, LJ, Granger LR, *et al.* (2008) National Athletic Trainers' Association position statement: preventing, detecting, and managing disordered eating in athletes. *J Athl Train*, 43(1), 80–108.

Drinkwater B, Loucks A, Sherman R, Sundgot-Borgen J, and Thompson R; International Olympic Committee Medical Commission Working Group Women in Sport. (2005) *Position Stand on the Female Athlete Triad*. Available at http://www.olympic.org/Documents/Reports/EN/en_report_917.pdf (accessed May 22, 2013).

Flament MF, Bissada H, and Spettigue W. (2012) Evidence-based pharmacotherapy of eating disorders. *Int J Neuropsychopharmacol*, 15(2), 189–207.

Lebrun CM. (2007) The female athlete triad: what's a doctor to do? *Curr Sports Med Rep*, 6(6), 397–404.

Nattiv A, Loucks AB, Manore MM, Sanborn CF, Sundgot-Borgen J, and Warren MP. (2007) American College of Sports Medicine position stand. The female athlete triad. *Med Sci Sports Exerc*, 39(10), 1867–1882.

O'Connor H and Caterson I. (2006) Weight loss and the athlete. In L Burke and V Deakin (eds), *Clinical Sports Nutrition* (3rd edn, pp. 135–174). McGraw-Hill Australia Pty Ltd, North Ryde.

Rankin JW. (2006) Making weight in sports. In L Burke and V Deakin (eds), *Clinical Sports Nutrition* (3rd edn, pp. 175–199). McGraw-Hill Australia Pty Ltd, North Ryde.

Skårderud F, Fladvad T, Garthe I, Holmlund H, and Engebretsen L. (2012) The malnourished athlete – guidelines for interventions. Den dårlig ernærte utøveren. Vektreduksjon, kroppsmodifikasjon og spiseforstyrrelser i toppidrett. Retningslinjer for holdning og handling. Oslo: Olympiatoppen. http://www.olympiatoppen.no/fagomraader/idrettsarnaering/Fagstoff/page6827.html (accessed on June 4, 2012)

Smolak L, Murnen SK, and Ruble AE. (2000) Female athletes and eating problems: a meta-analysis. *Int J Eat Disorder*, 27, 371–380.

Sundgot-Borgen J. (1994) Risk and trigger factors for the development of eating disorders in female elite athletes. *Med Sci Sports Exerc*, 26, 414–419.

Sundgot-Borgen J and Torstveit MK. (2004) Prevalence of eating disorders in elite athletes is higher than in the general population. *Clin J Sport Med*, 14(1), 25–32.

Torstveit MK, Rosenvinge J, and Sundgot- Borgen J. (2008) Prevalence of eating disorders and the predictive power of risk factor models in female elite athletes: a controlled study. *Scand J Med Sci Spor*, 18(1), 108–118.

Thompson RA and Sherman RT. (2010) *Eating Disorders in Sport* (pp. 284). Routledge, Taylor & Francis Group, New York.

Warren MP. (2011) Endocrine manifestations of eating disorders. *J Clin Endocrinol Metab*. 96(2), 333–343.

Zach KN, Smith Machin AL, and Hoch AZ. (2011) Advances in management of the female athlete triad and eating disorders. *Clin Sports Med*, 30(3), 551–573.

Zerbe KJ. (2007) Eating disorders in the 21st century: identification, management, and prevention in obstetrics and gynecology. *Best Pract Res Clin Obstet Gynaecol*, 21(2), 331–343.

Chapter 6
Bone health

Naama W. Constantini[1] and Constance M. Lebrun[2,3]

[1]Sport Medicine Center, Department of Orthopedic Surgery, The Hadassah-Hebrew University Medical Center, Jerusalem, Israel
[2]Department of Family Medicine, Faculty of Medicine and Dentistry, University of Alberta, Edmonton, Alberta, Canada
[3]Glen Sather Clinic, University of Alberta, Edmonton, Alberta, Canada

Bone health in the female athlete

This chapter will review what is currently known about bone health in the female athlete, including assessment techniques and various factors that impact bone health—both positively (such as exercise) and negatively (including the Female Athlete Triad) (Figure 6.1). Strategies for optimizing bone mineral density at all ages will be discussed.

Assessment of bone health

Bone is an active tissue composed of connective tissue fibers, as well as various proteins and calcium–phosphorus deposits, all of which give it strength and resistance to varying degrees of loads. The skeleton is comprised mainly of two types of bone tissues—dense bone tissue (*compact bone*), found primarily in the outer part of cylindrical long bones, and spongy bone tissue (*trabecular bone*) that includes many spaces that give it the appearance of a sponge. As bone ages, the amount of bone is decreased and the structural integrity of trabecular bone is impaired. In addition, cortical bone becomes more porous and thinner. These changes make the bone weaker and more likely to fracture (Figure 6.2).

The strength of the bone is the most important measure to its quality and is affected by a number of components:

(a) Bone mineral density (BMD)
(b) Bone size (geometry)
(c) Micro-architectural structure of the bone
(d) Collagen and other proteins (provide hardness and flexibility to the skeleton)
(e) Bone metabolism—the turnover rate of bone tissue

Bone density itself accounts for about 70% of bone strength, and below a certain threshold, it may lead to osteopenia or osteoporosis.

The World Health Organization (WHO) has defined *osteopenia* as BMD between 1.0 and 2.5 standard deviations (SD) below normal, and *osteoporosis* as below 2.5 SD. The *T*-score relates to the score as compared with a 30-year-old woman, while the *Z*-score compares a woman's results to those women of her own age. These definitions were developed for the evaluation and management of postmenopausal women with low bone density and are frequently used as decision points for initiation of treatment.

There are several methods for assessing bone density status. The most common methods in clinical practice and research today are as follows:

1 Dual X-ray absorptiometry (DXA)—This is a simple, reliable test, with high repeatability that is suitable for predicting osteoporotic fractures. It is the only test that has been validated for osteoporosis diagnosis. The main disadvantage of this method is that it does not reflect other important factors

The Female Athlete, First Edition. Edited by Margo L. Mountjoy.
© 2015 International Olympic Committee. Published 2015 by John Wiley & Sons, Inc.

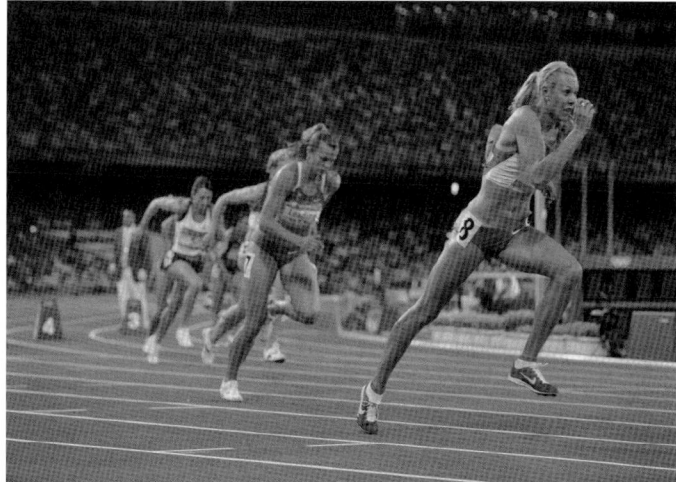

Figure 6.1 Normally, regular weight-bearing activity such as running is osteogenic. However, menstrual dysfunction associated with low energy availability may compromise optimal bone mineral density. Courtesy of the International Olympic Committee.

affecting bone strength, such as size, architecture, geometry, and elastic properties. Another drawback is it is actually a 2-dimensional measurement and therefore can be confounded by vertebral body size, and surrounding soft tissues leading to measurement errors.

2 Quantitative computed tomography (QCT)— This method allows 3-dimensional measurements of both trabecular bone and cortical bone, which assesses bone density with a greater accuracy than the DXA. The main disadvantages to this method are its low availability, high price, and the high radiation doses involved. Axial QCT is used for the spine and hip, while peripheral QCT (pQCT) can be used in the peripheral skeleton, such as the distal radius and tibia. The latter (pQCT) has a lower dose of radiation.

3 Quantitative ultra sound (QUS)—This technology is free of ionizing radiation, and is able to characterize important mechanical indices of bone (such as elasticity) that contribute to strength and resistance to fractures. Measurements are generally done at the calcaneus, generating two different parameters: the speed of sound (SOS) and broadband ultrasound attentuation (BUA). More sophisticated QUS indices can be derived from these two basic measures. The machines are compact and also relatively inexpensive. For these reasons, this assessment technique is sometimes used in initial screening for osteoporosis. There is a reasonable correlation with DXA, especially in postmenopausal women, but the correlation is not as good for predicting fractures. Another disadvantage is that QUS technology cannot measure the spine or hip, and it has lower repeatability; thus, it is not suitable for tracking changes over time.

Osteoporosis

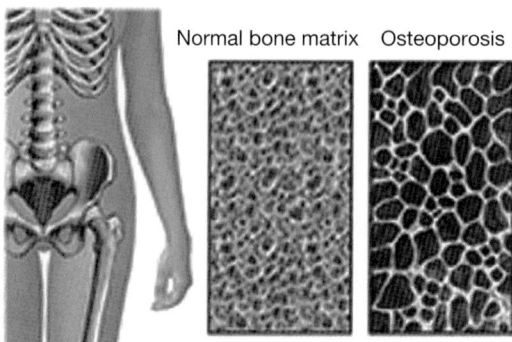

Figure 6.2 Diagram showing normal and osteoporotic bone. ©2013 Nucleus Medical Media, with permission.

Factors that impact bone health

Bone is a dynamic tissue. The acquisition of bone that occurs during childhood and adolescence accounts for 90% of adult bone mass. Bone mineral density is influenced by a number of intrinsic and extrinsic factors:

- Intrinsic factors:
  - **Genetics**—Between 60–90% of the variability in ultimate peak BMC is attributable to genetic factors. This also accounts for other bone health parameters such as bone geometry, bone turnover markers, and risk for osteoporotic fractures.
  - **Sex**—Women have lower BMD than men. Men however can also suffer from osteoporosis, under certain circumstances.
  - **Age**—BMD increases until the third decade and decreases gradually from the 5th decade of life onward in both sexes. There is an additional rapid decrease in the few years immediately during and after menopause, especially in trabecular bone (Figure 6.3).
  - **Body size**—People with low body weight and tiny bones have lower stimuli for bone mechanical loading and therefore lower BMD.
  - **Race and ethnicity**—White and Asian women have lower BMD as compared with Hispanic and African-American women.
  - **Family history** of osteoporosis and osteoporotic fractures is a strong predictor of low BMD and eventual fractures.
- Extrinsic (environmental) factors:
  - **Body weight**—Body mass index is correlated with BMD. Both lean body mass as well

as fat mass (which affects hormonal status, i.e., increases calcium absorption, reduces sensitivity to parathyroid hormone, etc.) have positive effects on bone density.

- **Diet**—**Calcium** and **vitamin D** are the most significant components in the diet that may affect bone mass. Other nutrients have been studied as having an effect of the bone status. These include dietary fibers, caffeine, alcohol, phosphorus, vitamin K, protein, sodium, and more.
  - Increased consumption of **dietary fibers** (over 30 grams per day) may interfere with the absorption of calcium, but this issue is considered negligible due to the relatively low fiber intake in the general population.
  - Daily consumption of beverages containing **caffeine** (several cups/day) may cause an increased loss of calcium in urine. Researchers do not agree about the effect of increased consumption of caffeine on bone density. Caffeine seems to have little impact, if any, on calcium and bone density in people who meet the daily calcium intake recommendations.
  - **Alcohol**—Increased consumption is a common cause of secondary osteoporosis through an increase in the incidence of fractures and complications in their recovery.
- **Exercise**—The specific effects of physical activity on bone health have been investigated in randomized clinical trials and observational studies. According to Wolff's law, bone reacts proportionally to the forces implied to it. The forces include compression forces from gravity, loads placed upon the bone with activity, and pulling forces at the tendon interface. Mechanical loading in childhood and during adolescence positively affects bone health in adulthood and decreases osteoporotic fractures, probably by increasing peak bone mass, whereas inactivity is associated with lower bone mass. Physical activity needs to be continuous throughout life in order to maintain the peak bone mass achieved and to prevent bone loss at any age.

The osteogenic effect of physical activity on bone is especially prominent in high-impact sports such as running, jumping, and ball games. On the other hand, swimming and cycling, which are non-impact sports (non-weight bearing) do not affect bone density much. The effect of physical activity

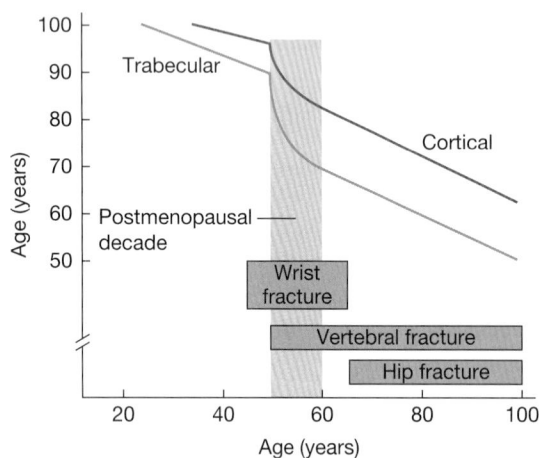

Figure 6.3 Schematic diagram showing changes in trabecular and cortical bone across the lifespan.

on bone mass depends also on the specific sites of impact of the various sport activities and therefore varies between bones. In tennis or squash players, for instance, upper extremity BMD is significantly higher on the dominant side compared with the nondominant side, especially if the athlete started playing at a younger age—premenarchal.

It appears that calcium intake especially during childhood, acts synergistically with physical activity to promote bone health, but physical activity has a larger osteogenic effect compared with calcium intake.

• **Sex hormones**—Sex steroids secreted during puberty substantially increase BMD and peak bone mass. Estrogen is osteoprotective, primarily through its action to inhibit bone resorption. It also facilitates Vitamin-D-related intestinal calcium absorption. Progesterone is thought by some researchers to have a role in stimulating bone formation. In adolescents and young women, the sustained production of estrogen is essential for the maintenance of bone mass. Reduction in estrogen production with menopause is the major cause of loss of BMD during later life. Timing of menarche (late menarche), absent or infrequent menstrual cycles, and the timing of menopause (early menopause) influence both the attainment of peak bone mass and the preservation of BMD. Testosterone has an anabolic effect on bone. Testosterone stimulates osteoblasts, and through its aromatization to estrogen, may also inhibit osteoclastic activity.

• **Other hormones**—Other important hormones for bone health include growth hormone (GH), IGF-1 (insulin-like growth factor-1), as well as leptin and other adipokines. Both GH and IGF-1 increase bone formation, and GH elevates the production of active form of vitamin D. Leptin regulates bone formation through both central (hypothalamic) and peripheral (direct) pathways, and leptin deficiency is associated with low bone mass.

• **Exercise and hormones**—There is a strong interaction between exercise and several reproductive hormones (estrogen, progesterone, testosterone), GH, IGF-1, stress hormones (catecholamines), and calciotropic hormones (PTH, calcitonin, vitamin D). In most cases, there is a synergistic, positive effect on the bone, whereas in some, especially with low energy intake, there is a negative effect.

• **Medications**—Drugs such as glucocorticosteroids, antiepileptics, and selective serotonin reuptake inhibitors (SSRIs), for example, decrease bone mass.

• **Smoking**—Cigarette smoking increases the risk of fractures in general, and osteoporotic fractures in particular in both men and women, mainly due to damage to bone density of the hip and spine. Several mechanisms have been proposed for this adverse effect of smoking on bone health, including injury to the micro-architectural structure of spongy bone, calcitonin resistance, lowered estrogen levels in smokers, decreased bone calcium sedimentation following elevated parathyroid hormone levels and an increase in bone breakdown among smokers.

• **Diseases**—Other diseases such as anorexia or bulimia nervosa, celiac or inflammatory bowel disease, or depression disease can adversely affect bone density. This may be through direct effects or due to medications used in treatment.

Bone health in female athletes

Maximal bone mass accrual occurs in females between 11 and 14 years of age and about 2–3 years later in males, with peak bone growth in both sexes around the time of the pubertal growth spurt. A recent longitudinal multicohort study of middle-class Caucasian females and males found that final peak bone mass occurred around 19 years in women and 20.5 years in men. No significant increase in bone mineral content was noted after that time point.

As stated in the previous section, peak bone mass is determined largely by genetic factors, with some 20–40% contributions from nutrition, endocrine status, physical activity, and health during growth. Weight-bearing sports and those with odd impacts are the most effective for increasing bone density, particularly before puberty. Higher BMD is reported in sports involving running, jumping, and weight lifting, and the positive effects have been shown to persist into adulthood. Not only is overall BMD improved, there are also substantial changes in bone geometry, with thicker cortices and therefore more cross-sectional strength and resistance to fracture.

If a female athlete does not reach her genetic potential for BMD, either through nutritional deprivation and/or by delayed menarche, and/or begins to lose BMD sooner than she should because of low energy availability and menstrual dysfunction, there is a possibility of reaching the threshold for fractures of the wrist, spine, and hip at a much earlier age. The associated morbidity and mortality is significant. Risk of fracture increases progressively with decreasing BMD, approximately twofold for each SD decrease in BMD, with a predictive value of BMD for hip fracture at least as good as that of blood pressure for stroke. Therefore, it is imperative that young female athletes optimize bone accrual during the prepubertal and adolescent years, and avoid bone resorption and loss of BMD.

To a certain extent, the osteogenic effect of weight-bearing exercise moderates the negative impact on BMD associated with menstrual dysfunction, but it is not completely protective. The permissive role of estrogen seems to be necessary for the bone anabolic effects of impact-loading exercise.

Optimal nutrition (calcium, vitamin D, but also overall adequate caloric intake) is necessary for the establishment of maximal bone mass. In female athletes, however, the greatest risk to BMD is menstrual dysfunction, including primary and secondary amenorrhea, oligomenorrhea, anovulatory cycles, and luteal phase deficiency. Amenorrhea and oligomenorrhea are relatively easy to monitor clinically, but subtle hormonal deficiencies associated with the latter two conditions can be difficult to detect. In any female athlete presenting with amenorrhea, it is critical to exclude other causes, such as pregnancy, polycystic ovarian syndrome (PCOS), pituitary tumor (prolactinoma), thyroid disorders, premature ovarian failure. Only then can the condition be labelled as functional hypothalamic amenorrhea (FHA). For athletes with amenorrhea, the duration of amenorrhea is associated with decreased bone density, and BMD is linked with the total lifetime number of ovulatory cycles. Athletes with amenorrhea have lower bone density not only in comparison with athletes with eumenorrhea, but also in comparison with nonathletic control subjects with normal menstruation. Therefore, in addition to the deleterious effects of amenorrhea

on bone health, some of the beneficial effects of exercise on bone density are actually being lost in girls who develop amenorrhea. Consequently, it is important to optimize both nutritional and menstrual status in athletes, in order to establish the maximal attainment of peak bone mass.

The female athlete triad

The Female Athlete Triad has been defined as the combination of three separate clinical entities—low energy availability (LEA) (with or without disordered eating), menstrual dysfunction, and low BMD. The WHO definitions for osteoporosis, as mentioned earlier in this chapter, were developed for the evaluation and management of postmenopausal women. Subsequently, the International Society for Clinical Densitometry has indicated that these categories are not relevant for premenopausal women (especially young women) or for men. Instead, Z-scores, but not T-scores, are preferred, and this is particularly important in children. A Z-score of -2.0 or lower is defined as "below the expected range for age," and a Z-score above -2.0 is "within the expected range for age." The American College of Sports Medicine (ACSM), in their 2007 position stand on the Female Athlete Triad, used a slightly different definition. They suggested that because athletes in weight-bearing sports should have 5–15% higher BMD than nonathletes, a BMD Z-score <-1.0 warrants further attention. "Low BMD" is defined as a Z-score between -1.0 and -2.0, together with a history of nutritional deficiencies, hypoestrogenism, stress fractures, and/or other secondary clinical risk factors for fracture. To reflect an increased risk of fragility fracture, ACSM defines "osteoporosis" as secondary clinical risk factors for fractures with BMD Z-scores $<= -2.0$. These differences in terminology and lack of universal screening for BMD have made it difficult to accurately estimate the overall prevalence of altered bone density in female athletes.

Examples of DXA scans in a young runner with the Female Athlete Triad are shown (Figures 6.4 and 6.5). In this case, she would be categorized as having "osteoporosis" by both WHO criteria and the ACSM definition, based on the DXA of her spine. Her femur BMD values are slightly higher, due to the protective effect of impact loading from her sport. However, the

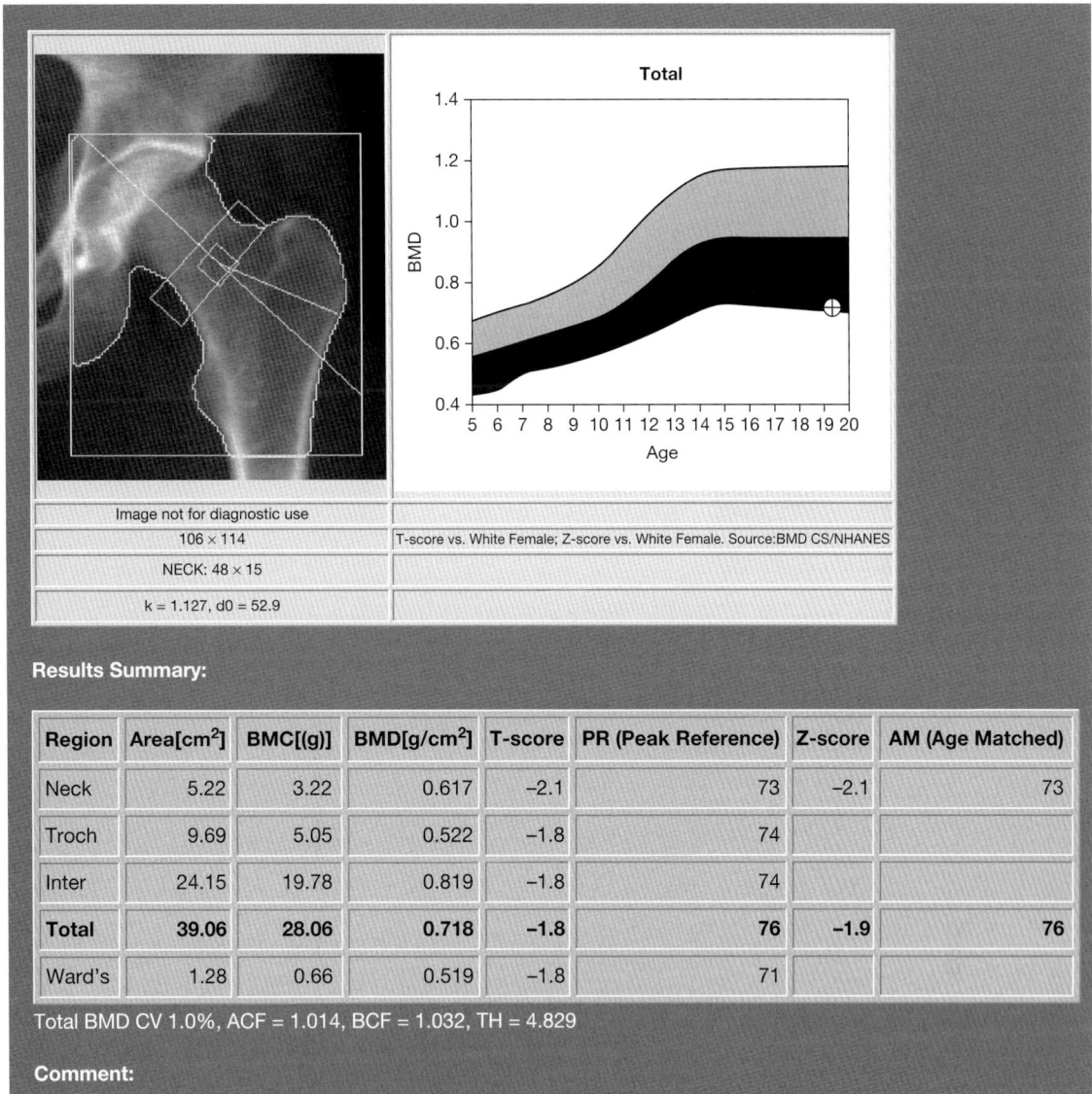

106 × 114

NECK: 48 × 15

k = 1.127, d0 = 52.9

T-score vs. White Female; Z-score vs. White Female. Source:BMD CS/NHANES

Results Summary:

Region	Area[cm^2]	BMC[(g)]	BMD[g/cm^2]	T-score	PR (Peak Reference)	Z-score	AM (Age Matched)
Neck	5.22	3.22	0.617	–2.1	73	–2.1	73
Troch	9.69	5.05	0.522	–1.8	74		
Inter	24.15	19.78	0.819	–1.8	74		
Total	**39.06**	**28.06**	**0.718**	**–1.8**	**76**	**–1.9**	**76**
Ward's	1.28	0.66	0.519	–1.8	71		

Total BMD CV 1.0%, ACF = 1.014, BCF = 1.032, TH = 4.829

Comment:

Figure 6.4 DXA scan of the femur in 19-year-old athlete with menstrual dysfunction and past history of an eating disorder.

BMD measurements of the spine reflect mainly trabecular bone and therefore give a better picture of her overall bone health status.

Biochemical markers of bone remodeling (e.g., resorption markers-serum C-telopeptide and urinary N-telopeptide, and formation markers-serum bone-specific alkaline phosphatase, osteocalcin (OC), and amino-terminal propeptide of type 1 procollagen) are sometimes used clinically to assess bone turnover, mostly in the setting of assessing response to treatment for osteoporosis in postmenopausal women. However, there may be some clinical benefit to using them in younger populations at risk of losing BMD. In some studies, lower bone density in athletes with amenorrhea was associated with lower levels of bone formation and bone-resorption markers, indicating a state of reduced bone turnover. Research has also shown

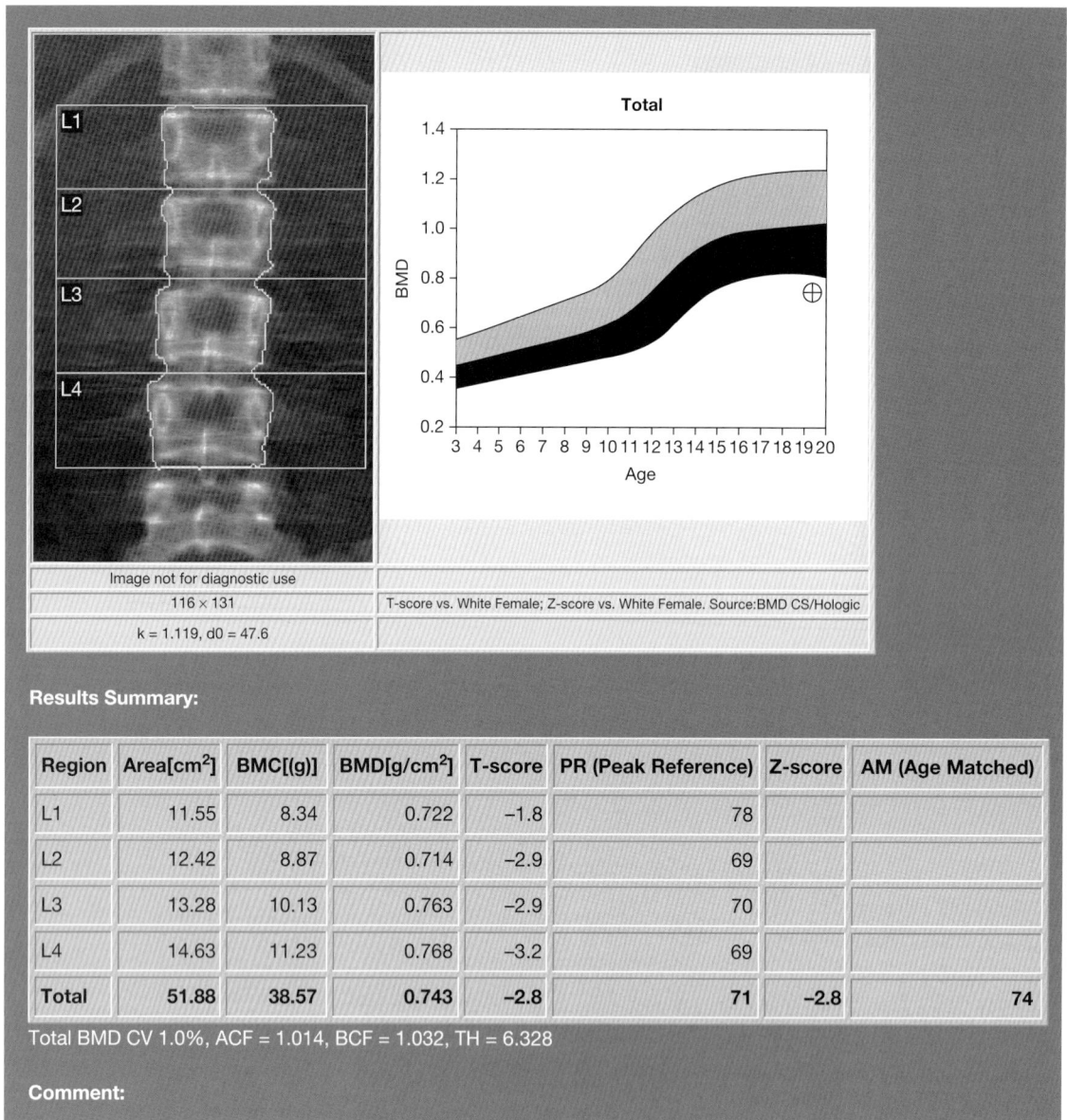

Region	Area[cm²]	BMC[(g)]	BMD[g/cm²]	T-score	PR (Peak Reference)	Z-score	AM (Age Matched)
L1	11.55	8.34	0.722	−1.8	78		
L2	12.42	8.87	0.714	−2.9	69		
L3	13.28	10.13	0.763	−2.9	70		
L4	14.63	11.23	0.768	−3.2	69		
Total	51.88	38.57	0.743	−2.8	71	−2.8	74

Total BMD CV 1.0%, ACF = 1.014, BCF = 1.032, TH = 6.328

Comment:

Figure 6.5 DXA scan of the spine in the same athlete.

a dose-dependent response of bone turnover to energy availability, with restricted energy availability impairing bone formation. When the restriction was severe enough to depress estradiol levels, then increased bone resorption also occurred.

Women with menstrual dysfunction are more prone to musculoskeletal injuries in general, and in particular, a two- to fourfold increase in stress fractures. These are injuries that occur with repetitive overloading and consequent microtraumas to the bone (Figure 6.6). The magnitude of the loading is not as great as it would need to be in women with normal BMD. Therefore, any female athlete presenting with a stress fracture, or fracture from minimal trauma, should also be asked about her menstrual history and her nutritional status.

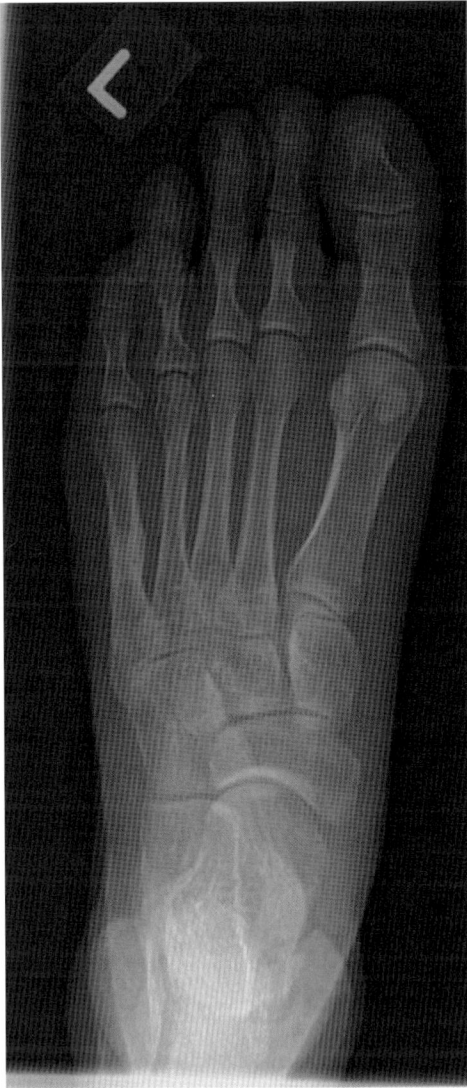

Figure 6.6 X-ray of left foot in the same athlete—incomplete stress fracture of 3rd metatarsal bone and healed stress fracture of 5th metatarsal.

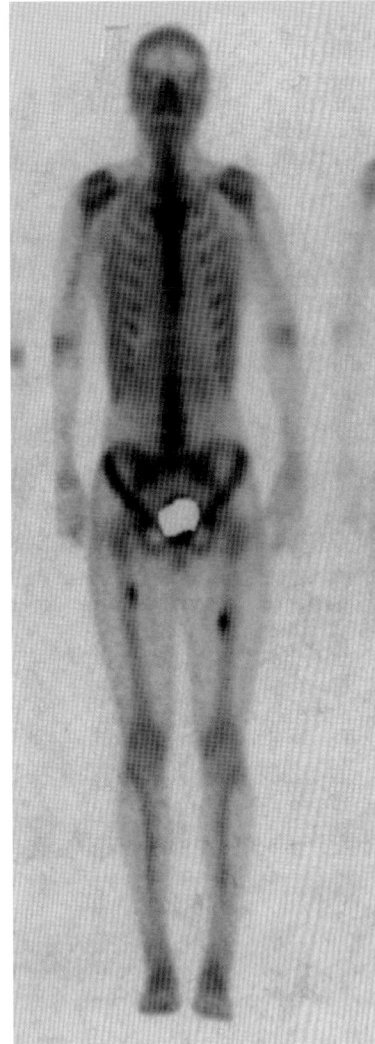

Figure 6.7 Bone scan showing bilateral stress fractures of the femur in a female distance runner.

Bone scans are helpful when initial radiographs are negative in the clinical setting of a probable stress fracture (Figure 6.7). In many cases, the actual stress fracture does not appear on plain radiographs until after it has healed (see Figure 6.6). Certain stress fractures (such as those in the navicular bone, or the femoral neck or shaft) are considered high risk and can go on to complete fracture (with significant consequences) if not recognized early and managed appropriately with restriction of weight-bearing activity and impact until healed.

Management to optimize bone health

Initial management rests on early identification of the problem of low BMD. Proper nutrition with adequate energy availability is the cornerstone in preventing bone loss and optimizing bone health.

In many cases, simple awareness of dietary inadequacies can be improved—as the female athlete may inadvertently not be replacing the energy used for physical activities. Simple strategies, such as increasing caloric intake by 300–500 Kcal/day, or decreasing activity by 10% may be enough to reverse the menstrual dysfunction and initiate menses again. A trial of 6–12 months of nonpharmacologic therapy is reasonable, with close monitoring of the athlete. Nutritional counselling by a trained professional is also of great benefit.

If low BMD has already been documented in a young female athlete, and/or if she has suffered one or more stress fractures, then there is more urgency in initiating pharmacologic measures. Calcium intake should reach 1000 mg/day for over 18 and 1300 mg/day for younger athletes and vitamin D 600–1000 I.U./day or even more depending on vitamin D level of deficiency. If dietary sources are poor, then supplementation should be considered. Vitamin D deficiency is common in northern climates, particularly in the winter, when there are less hours of sunlight per day. Other factors, such as dark skin, use of sunscreen, or spending excessive amounts of time indoors, are also contributory.

Oral hormone replacement therapies (HRT) including oral contraceptives (OC) are an artificial way to achieve "regular" menses but have not been proven to increase bone density or prevent bone loss in females suffering from anorexia nervosa or athletes with hypothalamic amenorrhea due to LEA. There are also no data that show that they reduce stress fractures. On the contrary, there are studies that show a negative effect on bone health, given the first-pass effects on hepatic production of insulin-like growth factor-1 (IGF-1), which is a bone formation hormone, and is low to start with in energy-deficient states. Moreover, HRT/OC give a false impression that the body has resumed normal function thus masking the number one red flag of LEA – amenorrhea.

There are some promising reports that transdermal estradiol administration, when given in replacement doses, does not suppress IGF-1 and therefore might be effective in preventing bone loss. However, these trials were done on adolescent girls with anorexia nervosa and so far no prospective, randomized, controlled study has examined the effect on athletes with FHA and low bone mass.

The effect of vaginal estradiol administration or the vaginal estrogen-progesterone combination contraceptive ring should also be investigated as both forms circumvent hepatic first-pass metabolism.

Female athletes with LEA who need contraception should consult a sport physician or a sport gynecologist for advice.

Bisphosphonates (such as alendronate, ibandronate, risedronate, etidronate, zoledronate) are analogs of inorganic pyrophosphate and inhibit resorption of bone and can therefore be useful in this older population. BMD increases after treatment with alendronate, etidronate and risedronate. However, for the most part, these drugs should not be used in women of reproductive age, as they are stored in bone for long periods of time (decades) and have been shown to be teratogenic. Adequate calcium intake is also necessary for them to be effective—in many cases calcium is combined with the active drug.

Other therapies in the postmenopausal age group include raloxifene (a selective estrogen receptor modulator or SERM) and parathyroid hormone (PTD) peptides. The latter have anabolic skeletal effects, most marked in cancellous bone. Teriparatide (recombinant human PTH 1-34) is available in North America, and recombinant human PTH (1-84) in Europe. Synthetic parathyroid hormone (PTH) makes theoretical sense and has been used in Paget's disease and in men with severe osteoporosis, but not in young women. It is a daily injectable medication, so compliance may be an issue.

Of note, raloxifene and other medications in the SERM class are actually prohibited substances on the list of the World Anti-Doping Agency. As such, it would be necessary to obtain a therapeutic use exemption (TUE), in order for the athlete to be able to use one of them. This requires an application to the relevant antidoping authority by the athlete's physician, including a complete medical history and rationale for use (stating whether other medications that are not on the prohibited list have been tried first). However, it is quite rare that these medications would be used in the younger athlete.

Calcitonin (administered in intranasal form) is an endogenous polypeptide hormone that inhibits osteoclastic bone resorption. It is primarily approved for the treatment of osteoporosis in women who are at least five years postmenopausal. There is very little research on its use in the younger female athlete with low BMD. Denusomab (RANKL inhibitor), strontium, and tibolone are all newer additional therapies for the treatment of osteoporosis. The latter two are only available in Europe. Strontium ranelate has a dual effect on bone remodeling, being able to stimulate bone formation by osteoblasts, a property shared with bone-forming agents, and to inhibit bone resorption by osteoclasts, as do anti-resorptive agents.

Other potential therapies are on the horizon, but large clinical trials are lacking. Insulin-derived growth factor (IGF-1) is a bone anabolic agent and has been found experimentally to normalize IGF-1 levels in anorexia. In combination with estrogen replacement therapy, it increases BMD in these patients. However, large-scale studies of its long-term safety and efficacy in treatment of osteoporosis in other clinical situations remains to be determined. Leptin, a hormonal mediator of adaptation to energy deprivation, is low in females with disordered eating and FHA. When given to this population, it leads to a beneficial effect on resumption of menses, and an associated increase in BMD. However, it may only be helpful in lean females who are low in leptin to start with.

In general, however, prevention is always better than any form of treatment. Optimal BMD in female athletes is maintained by weight-bearing exercise throughout the lifespan, adequate nutrition in terms of total calories, calcium and Vitamin D, and regular menstrual cycles with normal levels of estrogen and progesterone. Alterations from this ideal balance should be detected and managed expeditiously.

Acknowledgments

The authors wish to thank Ran Shabtai, a promising medical student, for his assistance in literature search and some writing.

Recommended reading

Barrack MT, Rauh MJ, Barkai HS, and Nichols JF. (2008) Dietary restraint and low bone mass in female adolescent endurance runners. *Am J Clin Nutr*, 87(1), 36–43.

Bass S, Pearce G, Bradney M, *et al.* (1998) Exercise before puberty may confer residual benefits in bone density in adulthood: studies in active prepubertal and retired female gymnasts. *J Bone Miner Res*, 13(3), 500–507.

Chilibeck PD. (2013) Hormonal regulations of the effects of exercise on bone: positive and negative effects. In N Constantini and AC Hackney (eds.) *Endocrinology of Physical Activity and Sport* (2nd edn, pp. 245–258). Contemporary Endocrinology Series, Humana Press, New York, NY.

Committee on Practice Bulletins-Gynecology, The American College of Obstetricians and Gynecologists. (2012) ACOG practice bulletin no. 129. Osteoporosis. *Obstet Gynecol*, 120(3), 718–734.

De Souza MJ, Nattiv A, Joy E, *et al.* (2014) 2014 the Female Athlete Triad Coalition Consensus Statement on Treatment and Return to Play of the Female Athlete Triad: 1st International Conference held in San Francisco, California, May 2012 and 2nd International Conference held in Indianapolis, Indiana May 2013. *Br J Sports Med*, 48(4), 289–309.

Ducher G, Turner AI, Kukuljan S, *et al.* (2011) Obstacles in the optimization of bone health outcomes in the Female Athlete Triad. *Sports Med*, 41(7), 587–607.

Duncan CS, Blimkie CJ, Cowell CT, Burke ST, Briody JN, and Howman-Giles R. (2002) Bone mineral density in adolescent female athletes: relationship to exercise type and muscle strength. *Med Sci Sports Exerc*, 34(2), 286–294.

Ginty F, Rennie KL, Mills L, Stear S, Jones S, and Prentice A. (2005) Positive, site-specific associations between bone mineral status, fitness, and time spent at high-impact activities in 16- to 18-year-old boys. *Bone*, 36(1), 101–110.

International Society for Clinical Densitometry Writing Group for the ISCD Position Development Conference. (2004) Diagnosis of osteoporosis in men, women, and children. *J Clin Dent*, 7(1), 17–26.

International Society for Clinical Densitometry. (2013) Official Positions. www.iscd.org. Updated August 15, 2013. http://www.iscd.org/official-positions./ (accessed on November 6, 2013).

Iuliano-Burns S, Stone J, Hopper JL, and Seeman E. (2005) Diet and exercise during growth have site-specific skeletal effects: a co-twin control study. *Osteoporos Int*, 16(10), 1225–1232.

Loud KJ, and Gordon CM. (2006) Adolescent bone health. *Arch Pediatr Adolesc Med*, 160(10), 1026–1032.

Mountjoy M, Sundgot-Borgen J, Burke L, *et al.* (2014) The IOC consensus statement: beyond the Female Athlete Triad–Relative Energy Deficiency in Sport (RED-S). *Br J Sports Med*, 48(7), 491–497.

Nattiv A, Loucks AB, Manore MM, Sanborn CF, Sundgot-Borgen J, and Warren MP. (2007) American College of Sports Medicine position stand: the Female Athlete Triad. *Med Sci Sports Exerc*, 39(10), 1867–1882.

Nilsson M, Ohlsson C, Eriksson AL, *et al.* (2008) Competitive physical activity early in life is associated with bone mineral density in elderly Swedish men. *Osteoporos Int*, 19(11), 1557–1566.

Small RE. (2005) Uses and limitations of bone mineral density measurements in the management of osteoporosis. *Med Gen Med*, 7(2), 3.

Valero C, Zarrabeitia MT, Hernandez JL, Zarrabeitia A, Gonzalez-Macias J, and Riancho JA. (2005) Bone mass in young adults: relationship with gender, weight and genetic factors. *J Intern Med*, 258(6), 554–562.

Van Langendonck L, Lefevre J, Claessens AL, *et al.* (2003) Influence of participation in high-impact sports during adolescence and adulthood on bone mineral density in middle-aged men: a 27-year follow-up study. *Am J Epidemiol*, 158(6), 525–533.

Chapter 7
Menstrual health in the female athlete

Madhusmita Misra

Pediatric Endocrine and Neuroendocrine Units, Massachusetts General Hospital and Harvard Medical School, Boston, MA, USA

Introduction

Menstrual dysfunction is a component of the Female Athlete Triad and is more commonly observed with certain kinds of athletic activities. This chapter will review normal menstrual function, causes and consequences of abnormal menstrual function in athletes, and management strategies for menstrual dysfunction.

What is normal puberty and normal menstrual function?

Pubertal onset and the hypothalamic–pituitary–gonadal axis: The hypothalamus secretes gonadotropin-releasing hormone (GnRH) is a pulsatile fashion, which then stimulates the secretion of follicle-stimulating hormone (FSH) and luteinizing hormone (LH) by the pituitary gland, and FSH and LH in turn stimulate secretion of estrogen and progesterone by the ovaries in girls. Puberty begins when the hypothalamic–pituitary–gonadal (HPG) axis awakens from its quiescent prepubertal state and is characterized by very specific changes in patterns of gonadotropin pulsatility. Early in puberty, GnRH pulsatility (reflected by LH pulsatility) changes from a prepubertal pattern of very low amplitude pulses to a pattern of nighttime increases in pulse amplitude, followed eventually by an increase in daytime pulsatility to approximate adult patterns. Factors that trigger pubertal onset are still under investigation; however, a withdrawal of inhibitory signals (such as GABA and neuropeptide YY) and an increase in excitatory signals (such as kisspeptin, glutamate, norepinephrine, and certain growth factors) have been implicated in this process. Nutritional signals are also key to pubertal onset. Although there is no threshold body weight or fat mass above which pubertal onset occurs, it is likely that a genetically determined threshold exists for any single individual for puberty to begin and progress. Proposed endocrine, metabolic, and nutritional signals for pubertal onset and progression include leptin, ghrelin, insulin, insulin-like growth factor-1 (IGF-1), galanin-like peptide, glucose, and free fatty acids.

Pubertal changes and their timing: During puberty, increasing estradiol secretion from ovarian follicles causes the development of secondary sexual characteristics, namely enlargement of breasts and the uterus. Breast development in girls heralds the onset of puberty (Tanner stage 2), and typically begins between 8 and 13 years of age. Rising levels of estradiol are followed by increases in growth hormone (GH) and IGF-1, which cause the pubertal growth spurt. In girls, growth velocity peaks at Tanner stage 3 of puberty. With further maturation of gonadotropin pulsatility and increasing secretion of gonadal steroids, menses begin, usually toward the end of Tanner stage 4 of puberty. In healthy girls, menarche, or the onset of menses, occurs 2–3 years after the onset of breast development and between 10 and 15 years of age. The average age for menarche is 12.7 years (SD 1.3 years) for girls in the United States, and minor racial and ethnic differences are reported. Cycles are often anovulatory, and hence, irregular for a variable period following menarche as the positive feedback effect of estradiol on the HPG axis is yet to be established. Over time, a larger proportion of cycles become ovulatory, leading to a more regular pattern of menstrual cyclicity.

Puberty is considered to have occurred early if breast and pubic hair development begin before 8 years, and delayed if these begin after 13 years. Menarche is considered **delayed** if menses does not occur within 2–3 years of starting breast development or by 15 years of age. Lack of any menses at 16 years despite otherwise normal pubertal development is referred to as **primary amenorrhea**. In contrast, amenorrhea that occurs after a period of normal or near normal menses is referred to as **secondary amenorrhea**. The duration of absent menses to qualify for secondary amenorrhea remains a matter of debate and ranges from 3 to 6 months.

Normal menstrual cycle: In the early follicular phase, increasing secretion of FSH causes enlargement and maturation of secondary ovarian follicles into antral follicles, proliferation of granulosa cells, induction of aromatase activity, and increased expression of FSH receptors on granulosa cells. Theca cells are evident as a layer of cells around the granulosa cells in the preantral stage, and secrete androgens in response to LH. Cross-talk between the theca and granulosa cells and aromatization of androgens (produced in theca cells) to estrogens within the granulosa cells lead to high levels of estrogen within the follicle. Rising estradiol levels cause thickening of the endometrial lining of the uterus with proliferation of stroma and uterine glands, and elongation of spiral arterioles. This is the proliferative phase of the uterine endometrium, corresponding with the follicular phase of the cycle.

Increasing estradiol secretion in the follicular phase then causes inhibition of FSH secretion by negative feedback. This allows selection of a dominant follicle, as smaller follicles that are still FSH dependent for growth become atretic. Increasing estradiol secretion from the dominant follicle around mid-cycle triggers the mid-cycle LH surge, followed by ovulation.

In the second half of the menstrual cycle, granulosa cells become luteinized and secrete progesterone. This is the luteal phase, and progesterone levels typically peak around day 21 of the cycle. Rising progesterone levels stabilize the endometrium and prepare it for implantation by a fertilized embryo. The granulosa cells of the corpus luteum also secrete inhibin, which inhibits FSH secretion and prevents growth of other follicles. If fertilization of the oocyte does not occur, there is eventual regression of the corpus luteum, a decrease in levels of estrogen and progesterone and constriction of the spiral arterioles, followed by shedding of the uterine lining as menses. The period between ovulation and menses is the luteal phase of the menstrual cycle, which corresponds to the secretory phase of the uterine lining. A gradual increase in FSH then heralds the onset of the next menstrual cycle.

Cycle length and menstrual flow: During the adolescent years, cycle length ranges between 20 and 45 days, and decreases to 24–38 days with increasing maturity. Cycle length longer than 45 days indicates **oligomenorrhea** and requires evaluation. In adolescents, 60–80% of cycles are between 21 and 35 days long by the third postmenarchal (gynecologic) year. While anovulatory cycles are more likely to be associated with short- or long-cycle length, there is a significant overlap with ovulatory cycles. The absence of premenstrual symptoms and dysmenorrhea suggests anovulatory cycles. Earlier menarche has been associated with earlier establishment of regular ovulatory cycles. Some women have ovulatory cycles with a short luteal phase, referred to as luteal phase dysfunction. The latter may be a cause of infertility or frequent miscarriages.

Menstrual flow typically lasts between 2 and 7 days and average blood loss during menses is about 30 mL in an adult. Consistent menstrual blood loss in excess of 80 mL can cause anemia. **Menorrhagia** refers to blood flow that is excessive and/or lasts longer than 7 days. Please see Table 7.1 for questions to ask to elicit a complete menstrual history.

Table 7.1 Questions to elicit menstrual history of an adolescent

How old were you when you had your first period?

Do you remember more specifically?—[*prompting*] Was it winter or summer? Were you closer to 12 or 13 or somewhere in between?

Do you write down the dates of your periods?

Do your periods come about once a month?

Have you ever skipped a month?

What is the longest you have gone without a period?

How many days do your periods typically last?

Would you describe your periods as light, medium, or heavy?

Do you typically use tampons or pads?

Have you ever used tampons?

Do you regularly use tampons?

Any difficulty in using tampons?

On a typical day, how many times a day do you have to change a tampon or a pad? Think about from the time you get up in the morning, the number of times you change at school, and then the number of times you change after you get home from school.

If bleeding described as heavy:

Do you ever have accidents? Messing up panties or clothes or sheets?

Can you go all night without getting up to change?

Do you ever have to wear a tampon and a pad together?

Do you have cramps or pain with your periods?

Primary dysmenorrhea is suggested by onset cramps with the onset of bleeding or slightly before; worst pain day 1 or 2, pain that typically is not severe throughout the bleeding

Do you have any other symptoms with your periods?

Headaches?

Bloating?

Breast tenderness?

Anything else?

Do you miss school or have to change your plans because of your periods?

Is it because of how heavy they are?

Is it because of pain?

Is it because of other symptoms?

Source: Reproduced with permission from Adams Hillard (2008).

Causes of menstrual dysfunction

While a complete description of the causes and work-up of menstrual dysfunction is beyond the scope of this chapter, these include (i) heavy bleeding (menorrhagia), (ii) irregular bleeding, and (iii) amenorrhea. **Heavy bleeding** may occur in the years following menarche and often resolves spontaneously over time. Other causes include (a) bleeding, coagulation, and platelet disorders (including von Willebrand disease and idiopathic thrombocytopenic purpura), (b) thyroid dysfunction, (c) hyperprolactinemia and PCOS (associated with anovulatory cycles), (d) fibromyomas and adenomyosis, or (e) dysfunctional uterine bleeding. Evaluation should focus on these possible causes of menorrhagia and should include an assessment of hematocrit and iron studies to determine the need for iron supplementation.

Irregular bleeding includes oligomenorrhea (infrequent irregular cycles) and frequent episodes of irregular bleeding. Oligomenorrhea and amenorrhea are often collectively termed oligoamenorrhea, which can have hypogonadotropic or hypergonadotropic causes. Primary amenorrhea also needs to be worked up for **eugonadotropic** causes, such as an absent or hypoplastic uterus or cervix, and noncanalization of the cervix and/or vagina. A history of cyclic abdominal pain without menses is suggestive of bleeding into the uterus without egress because of a noncanalized cervix or vagina. If only the hymen is closed, the physical examination reveals a bulging bluish hymen from collection of menstrual blood in the vagina. Higher levels of noncanalization may require an internal examination, and imaging studies such as a sonogram or MRI are usually diagnostic. Polycystic ovarian syndrome (PCOS) may sometimes manifest as primary amenorrhea, but usually manifests as secondary amenorrhea. PCOS is suspected when there is evidence of clinical hyperandrogenism (hirsutism beyond that expected for race and ethnicity, excessive acne, temporal balding) and after ruling out pregnancy, merits assessment of gonadotropin and androgen levels (testosterone, free or bioavailable testosterone, DHEAS, 8 AM 17-hydroxy progesterone). Evidence of virilization (clitoromegaly, change in voice), with elevated androgens and androgen precursors (DHEA, DHEAS, and 8 AM 17-hydroxy progesterone) should raise concerns for late onset CAH and androgen-secreting tumors. It is always important to rule out pregnancy as a cause of amenorrhea.

Hypergonadotropic hypogonadism (GnRH independent) is associated with elevations in gonadotropins, particularly FSH, above the normal range, and indicates ovarian insufficiency. This is seen in the following:

(i) chromosomal disorders such as Turner syndrome and gonadal dysgenesis,

(ii) other causes of premature ovarian insufficiency such as fragile X premutations and autoimmune ovarian failure,

(iii) exposure of the ovaries to radiation or to alkylating chemotherapeutic agents, and

(iv) conditions such as galactosemia and mumps oophoritis.

The history and physical examination may suggest the diagnosis. Consistently elevated FSH levels drawn two weeks apart are diagnostic of a hypergonadotropic state. If the history is not contributory,

a karyotype and further genetic studies are often necessary. Because of the known clustering of autoimmune conditions, patients with a presumptive diagnosis of autoimmune disease should also be assessed for primary adrenal insufficiency and followed regularly by an endocrinologist.

Hypogonadotropic hypogonadism (GnRH dependent) is associated with low or low normal levels of gonadotropins with impaired pulsatility patterns. Common causes include the following:

(i) Functional hypothalamic amenorrhea as seen in patients with low-weight eating disorders, in exercise-induced amenorrhea (heavy exercisers, dancers, and certain athletes), depressive disorders, and chronic systemic disease

(ii) Hyperprolactinemia from a prolactinoma, medications causing prolactin elevations (such as risperidone, other antipsychotics, and metoclopramide), and severe hypothyroidism

(iii) Pituitary and extrapituitary tumors, infection, and infiltrative processes

(iv) Genetic causes (idiopathic hypogonadotropic hypogonadism caused by mutations in *KAL-1, FGFR-1, FGF-8, PROK2, PROKR2, NELF, TAC3, TAC3R, and CHRG* genes, and transcription factor defects causing multiple pituitary hormone deficiencies such as mutations in *PROP-1, LHX3, LHX4* genes)

The history and physical examination is usually revealing. Laboratory evaluation should include a pregnancy test, levels of gonadotropins, gonadal steroids (estradiol and testosterone), prolactin, TSH, and free T4 levels.

Menstrual function in the athlete and its determinants

Menstrual function in the athlete can range from normal ovulatory cycles to luteal phase defects, anovulatory cycles, oligomenorrhea, and complete amenorrhea. One study in teenage athletes reported oligoamenorrhea in up to 24% of all athletes. In older athletes, this can range from 3% to 66%. Even normally cycling exercisers may have underlying menstrual dysfunction. One study of recreational runners reported anovulatory cycles and luteal phase dysfunction in 12% and 43% of the women, compared with 0% and 10% of sedentary controls.

Menstrual status depends on multiple factors. These include the nature of athletic activity, the duration and intensity of training, and the athlete's nutritional status. Endurance sports such as long-distance track events, cross-country, swimming and cycling, and sports such as gymnastics and dancing are particularly associated with a higher risk of menstrual dysfunction. In addition, longer hours of training, lower body weight, disordered eating behaviors, greater dietary restraint, and greater drive for thinness are concerning for a greater risk for menstrual dysfunction. Overall, these factors translate to lower net energy availability, which depends on both energy intake and expenditure, and has been defined as [(Energy intake – Exercise energy expenditure)/Lean body mass].

Why is menstrual function disrupted in certain athletes? Menstrual function may be disrupted from all causes common to nonathletes (see ***Causes of menstrual dysfunction***). However, in athletes with oligoamenorrhea, after ruling out other causes, it is important to consider the diagnosis of functional hypothalamic amenorrhea or exercise-induced amenorrhea (a diagnosis of exclusion). When energy intake keeps pace with energy expenditure, normal menstrual function is typically maintained. However, when energy intake is insufficient to keep pace with energy expenditure, the body and the brain sense a state of net energy deficit, which then results in varying degrees of menstrual dysfunction. From an evolutionary perspective, in this state of energy deficit, energy is conserved for the most vital of body functions. The reproductive axis is presumably shut down as energy availability is insufficient to meet the energy needs of reproduction.

An important indicator of energy stores is body fat. Even among the athletes of normal weight, those who are amenorrheic have significantly lower body fat than eumenorrheic athletes, although there is a significant overlap across groups. It is thus possible that a genetically determined threshold or "set point" exists of energy availability (or body fat) for each individual above which normal menstrual function is permitted, and below which there is a

risk for menstrual dysfunction. Several hormones have been proposed as messengers of low energy availability/lower body fat that in turn impact the HPG axis. These include hormones secreted by fat such as leptin and adiponectin, and others regulated by energy status and body fat content, such as cortisol, ghrelin, peptide YY, insulin, and IGF-1.

Adipokines and the HPG axis: Adipokines are hormones secreted by adipocytes, such as leptin and adiponectin. Leptin has stimulatory effects on the HPG axis, and leptin levels decrease when fat mass decreases. Leptin levels are lower in amenorrheic athletes compared with normally menstruating athletes and nonathletes, and lower leptin levels predict lower LH pulse frequency and amplitude. Administration of recombinant human leptin to women with hypothalamic amenorrhea improves LH pulsatility with resumption of menses in up to 70% of women and resumption of ovulatory cycles in up to 40%. However, leptin is an anorexigenic hormone, and leptin administration causes reductions in appetite and weight loss in these women. Even when leptin dosing is adjusted to maintain weight, fat mass decreases in women who receive leptin. Thus, at this time, leptin administration is not a therapeutic option for amenorrheic athletes. In contrast to leptin, adiponectin levels increase with reductions in fat mass. Adiponectin inhibits gonadotropin secretion, and higher adiponectin levels associated with lower fat mass in amenorrheic athletes may also contribute to impaired gonadotropin pulsatility.

Hormones regulated by energy status and the HPG axis: Many gut and pancreatic hormones, such as ghrelin, peptide YY (PYY), and insulin, and hormones such as cortisol change with energy status and affect the HPG axis. Ghrelin is an appetite-inducing hormone secreted by the stomach, while PYY is an anorexigenic hormone secreted by the distal gut. Both hormones have inhibitory effects on gonadotropin secretion. In conditions of low fat mass, including in amenorrheic athletes, ghrelin and PYY levels increase, while insulin and IGF-1 levels decrease, all of which contribute to and predict reductions in gonadotropins. In addition, increases in cortisol, a gluconeogenic hormone, impact gonadotropin secretion adversely. Higher cortisol, ghrelin, and PYY, and lower insulin and IGF-1 levels in amenorrheic athletes predict impaired gonadotropin pulsatility and lower gonadotropin secretion. Data are lacking regarding effects of reducing availability of (or inhibiting action of) cortisol, ghrelin, and PYY, or of replacing IGF-1 on the HPG axis.

What are the consequences of menstrual dysfunction, particularly oligoamenorrhea?

Menstrual dysfunction in athletes is concerning (i) because it may indicate pathology that requires diagnosis and treatment and (ii) because of possible consequences of anovulation and/or oligoamenorrhea. If a specific pathological process is contributing to menstrual dysfunction, this needs to be diagnosed and treated. A complete history and physical examination should be performed followed by appropriate laboratory work-up. After ruling out pathological causes, concerns relate to the consequences of menstrual dysfunction. These include an impact on sexual function, uterine health, fertility, bone health, and potentially on cognitive measures, anxiety, and mood. When the cause of menstrual dysfunction is low energy availability from excessive exercise without sufficient caloric intake, the first line of management is non-pharmacological and aimed at increasing caloric intake and/or reducing exercise activity. Subsequently, replacement of gonadal hormones may be a consideration.

Impact on sexual function: Hypothalamic amenorrhea associated with low estrogen levels can cause vaginal dryness and dyspareunia, which typically responds well to (i) moisturizers and lubricants, and also to (ii) low-dose topical estrogen treatment (after ruling out contraindications for estrogen treatment such as estrogen-dependent tumors). Low-dose vaginal estrogen creams contain ≤50 mcg estradiol or ≤0.3 mg conjugated estrogens/≤0.5 g of the cream.

Impact on uterine health: An important question is whether inducing intermittent endometrial shedding is necessary to maintain uterine health in athletes with menstrual dysfunction. Therefore,

should oligoamenorrheic athletes be provided hormonal therapies that allow them to have intermittent menses? Unless the cause of oligoamenorrhea is PCOS, inducing endometrial shedding is usually not necessary. In PCOS, unopposed estrogen secretion leads to endometrial hyperplasia, which is the long run increases the risk for endometrial cancer. However, endometrial hyperplasia is unlikely in conditions of functional hypothalamic amenorrhea, where estrogen levels are low. Thus, hormonal therapy (either short courses of cyclic progesterone or cyclic estrogen/progesterone combination pills) to induce intermittent endometrial shedding and maintain uterine health is typically not necessary in exercise-induced oligoamenorrhea.

Impact on fertility: Anovulatory cycles and/or oligoamenorrhea in female athletes can result in infertility. Because this is a state of hypogonadotropic hypogonadism, the condition is usually reversible following reversal of the state of low energy availability, when HPG axis function normalizes. When reversal is incomplete or difficult to attain, assisted reproductive techniques are usually successful in inducing fertility. These include the use of clomifene, combinations of recombinant human FSH and human chorionic gonadotropin, or pulsatile GnRH using a pump.

Impact on bone: The greatest and most deleterious impact of hypogonadism in the female athlete is on bone health. In normal-weight athletes who are eumenorrheic, bone mineral density (BMD) is preserved and may even be higher than in nonathletes, particularly at cortical weight-bearing sites such as the hip. Although mechanical loading is beneficial for bone, this positive effect of mechanical loading is reduced when there is concurrent amenorrhea. Both adult and teenage amenorrheic athletes are at risk for low areal BMD (as assessed by dual-energy X-ray absorptiometry), particularly at predominantly trabecular sites such as the lumbar spine. Additionally, the beneficial effect of mechanical loading at the hip is lost in amenorrheic athletes, who have lower BMD at the hip than eumenorrheic athletes.

Studies of bone microarchitecture using high-resolution peripheral quantitative computed tomography have allowed the assessment of bone geometry and volumetric BMD in athletes and an understanding of geometric parameters that impact bone strength. At the non-weight-bearing sites, amenorrheic athletes compared with nonathletes have lower trabecular volumetric BMD and lower measures of stiffness and failure load (surrogates for bone strength as assessed by finite element analysis). At weight-bearing sites, amenorrheic athletes have reduced percent cortical area, increased trabecular separation, and lower trabecular number and total volumetric BMD. As a consequence, they lose the beneficial effects of mechanical loading on bone strength observed in eumenorrheic athletes at these sites. Amenorrheic athletes are at a higher risk overall for stress and nonstress fractures than eumenorrheic athletes.

The primary hormonal determinant of low BMD in athletes is hypogonadism, and older menarchal age and a longer duration of amenorrhea are both important contributors. Other hormonal factors include relatively lower IGF-1 and leptin and relatively higher cortisol, ghrelin, and PYY (seen in amenorrheic compared with eumenorrheic athletes and nonathletes), as well as coincidental hyperthyroidism and hyperparathyroidism. Other predisposing factors include lower BMI and lean body mass, vitamin D deficiency, and malabsorptive states. Repetitive impact (long-distance running and cross-country) confers a greater risk for low BMD in the amenorrheic state than high/odd impact. Mild forms of osteogenesis imperfecta may need to be considered in those with debilitating fractures after ruling out other causes for low BMD.

Please refer to the chapter on Bone Density in Athletes for details regarding who should undergo bone density testing, and non-pharmacological as well as pharmacological approaches to improve bone health. Overall, the best strategy to improve bone health in athletes is to optimize nutritional and gonadal status. Optimizing energy availability by ensuring that caloric intake meets the energy needs of athletic activity is essential to normalizing menstrual status, which in turn is key to optimizing bone health. Calcium and vitamin D intake should be optimized in all athletes. Those with low vitamin D levels should undergo vitamin D replacement with the goal to maintain 25(OH)D levels in the range of 32–50 ng/mL (80–125 nmol/L). Data for oral estrogen treatment are conflicting in athletes and exercisers. However, physiologic estrogen replacement using the 100 mcg 17β-estradiol transdermal patch with cyclic progesterone has been shown to be effective in improving BMD in adolescent girls with anorexia nervosa, and studies of transdermal versus oral estradiol are ongoing in normal-weight amenorrheic athletes. Other medications should be considered only in conjunction with an endocrinologist or other specialist in metabolic bone diseases in special circumstances.

Impact on cognitive measures, anxiety, and mood: Although data are limited in athletes, studies in anorexia nervosa, another condition of very low energy availability, indicate that normalizing estrogen levels improves measures of cognitive function in adult women with the disorder. In addition, physiologic estrogen replacement improves anxiety measures in adolescent girls with anorexia nervosa. Furthermore, lower testosterone levels in women with anorexia nervosa have been associated with symptoms of anxiety and depression. These data put together suggest a role for gonadal hormone replacement in normalizing cognitive function, anxiety, and mood in hypogonadal states. However, more studies are necessary to confirm these findings.

Impact on muscle perfusion: A few studies have implicated hypogonadism as a cause for impaired muscle perfusion in exercising women. One study has shown that estrogen–progesterone combination pills are effective in improving endothelial function in exercisers, as measured by flow-mediated dilatation of the brachial artery. More studies are, however, necessary to determine the impact of hypogonadism on muscle perfusion in athletes.

When should an athlete consult with her care provider regarding her menses? When should her care provider discuss menstrual history?

Any athlete with a history of infrequent, absent, or scanty menses should consult with her care provider about her symptoms. However, any history of menstrual dysfunction should prompt a consultation. Thus, excessive bleeding during cycles or frequent cycles should also prompt an evaluation. Likewise, care providers should ask specific questions pertaining to menstrual status at every visit. These include age at menarche, frequency of cycles, duration of menses, periods of oligoamenorrhea in relation to training season and nutritional status, the last menstrual period, and the date for the previous menstrual period.

Evaluation of menstrual dysfunction

The work-up for menstrual dysfunction includes a detailed history and physical examination to rule out causes other than the Female Athlete Triad causing abnormal menses. Please see the section on **Causes of menstrual dysfunction** and also Table 7.1 (for questions to evaluate menstrual function and causes of menstrual dysfunction). Laboratory evaluation of oligoamenorrhea should include the following:

(a) a pregnancy test,

(b) levels of gonadotropins (to assess whether hypogonadism is gonadotropin dependent or independent),

(c) levels of estradiol, total and free testosterone (to rule of PCOS), DHEA and DHEAS (in patients with hyperandrogenic features to rule out adrenal tumors), 8 AM 17-OH progesterone (if late onset CAH is a concern),

(d) prolactin (to rule out hyperprolactinemia-causing hypogonadism),

(e) TSH and free T4 levels (to rule out thyroid dysfunction),

(f) karyotype (in those with elevated gonadotropins), and

(g) blood count, sedimentation rate, electrolytes, renal and liver function.

Additional testing may be necessary based on the history and physical examination, and results of initial testing. Testing for withdrawal bleeding following a short course of progesterone (5 mg medroxyprogesterone acetate BID for 5–10 days) is a good test of estrogen status. Withdrawal bleeding is unlikely when the uterine lining has not been previously primed by endogenous/exogenous estrogen. Lack of withdrawal bleeding following a course of progesterone thus helps differentiate hypogonadal conditions from PCOS. Administration of a combination of estrogen and progesterone for about three weeks is usually sufficient to build up enough endometrium in hypogonadal states to induce withdrawal bleeding.

How is oligoamenorrhea treated?

Nonpharmacological measures: As previously discussed, nonpharmacological approaches to treat oligoamenorrhea include optimizing nutritional intake, reducing activity level or both. A sports dietician should be consulted when it is important to optimize nutritional intake. Factors to consider include diet quality, timing of meals and snacks, and incorporation of energy dense foods into the daily schedule, particularly around times of intense activity.

Pharmacological measures: Hormone replacement strategies should be considered when hypogonadism is associated with sequelae such as dyspareunia, infertility, or very low bone density with a clinically significant history of fractures. Specific strategies for hormone replacement in these conditions have been discussed under the appropriate headings.

Contraception in the female athlete

Contraceptive options include all options available for nonathletes with similar risks and benefits. However, certain factors to be considered in athletes are as follows:

• Depot medroxyprogesterone acetate has a black box warning with respect to its deleterious effects on bone density. Thus, it may not be an optimal long-term contraceptive approach for athletes at risk for low bone density.

• Progesterone containing intrauterine devices (IUDs) may cause irregular menses and amenorrhea. This can make it challenging to determine whether an athlete is oligo-amenorrheic from reduced energy availability or from the IUD.

• Estrogen–progesterone containing oral contraceptive pills are not effective at improving bone density measures. Regular cycles on oral contraceptive pills may mask underlying menstrual dysfunction and may falsely reassure providers and athletes that hormone replacement in this form is helping bone health.

Conclusion

Menstrual health in the female athlete depends greatly on her state of energy availability. After pathological causes for menstrual dysfunction are ruled out, functional hypothalamic amenorrhea is usually an indication of inadequate caloric intake to meet energy expenditure needs. Consequences of functional hypothalamic amenorrhea include dyspareunia, infertility, and impaired bone health, and there are emerging data regarding a potential impact on muscle perfusion and function, and on neurocognitive health. Management includes ruling out other causes of menstrual dysfunction, and optimizing energy availability. Specific treatment strategies depend on the consequence of menstrual dysfunction that requires treatment.

Reference

Adams Hillard PJ. (2008) Menstruation in adolescents. *Ann N Y Acad Sci*, 1135, 29–35.

Recommended reading

Ackerman KE and Misra M. (2011) Bone health and the female athlete triad in adolescent athletes. *Phys Sports Med*, 39(1):131–141.

Misra M. (2012) Effects of hypogonadism on bone metabolism in adolescent and young adult women. *Nat Rev Endocrinol*, 8(7):395–404.

Misra M, Katzman DK, Miller KK, *et al.* (2011) Physiologic estrogen replacement increases bone density in adolescent girls with anorexia nervosa. *J Bone Miner Res*, 26(10):2430–2438.

The Menstrual Cycle and Adolescent Health. (2008) Eds: Gordon CM, Welt C, Rebar RW, Hillard PJA, Matzuk MM, Nelson LM. The Menstrual Cycle and Adolescent Health (Annals of the New York Academy of Sciences: Volume 1135), Wiley-Blackwell, New York, NY.

Chapter 8
Exercise and pelvic floor dysfunction in female elite athletes

Kari Bø

Department of Sports Medicine, Norwegian School of Sport Sciences, Oslo, Norway

Pelvic floor anatomy, function, and dysfunction

The pelvic floor muscles (PFM) forms the bottom of the pelvis and the floor of the abdominal cavity. They comprise a three-layer muscle plate with two mayor muscle groups: the pelvic and the urogenital diaphragm. The area surrounding the pelvic openings in women (the urethra, vagina, and the anus) bordering the medial layer of the muscles on both sides is named levator hiatus and is the largest hernia port in the body. The PFM is the only muscle group in the body capable of giving structural support for the pelvic organs, and during contraction, the pelvic openings are narrowed preventing leakage of urine, flatus, or stool. Correct contraction of the PFM has been described as a squeeze around the pelvic openings (a 25% narrowing of the levator hiatus area has been measured on ultrasound) and a forward/inward lift of the muscles (a lift of approximately 1 cm has been measured on ultrasound).

Unfortunately, some women are not able to contract the PFM correctly, and several studies from different countries have found that more than 30% of pregnant women, and women with pelvic floor dysfunction, may not be able to contract correctly at their first consultation. Common errors are to use gluteal hip adductors and abdominal muscles instead of the PFM, and one study found that 25% of women were straining instead of squeezing and lifting. Pushing down/straining might further weaken and stretch the PFM, and pushing is a risk factor for the development of pelvic organ prolapse. Proper teaching and assessment of ability to perform a correct contraction is therefore necessary before starting a PFM training (PFMT) program. Lack of an automatic, unconscious co-contraction or delayed or weak co-contraction of the PFM may lead to urinary incontinence, fecal incontinence, and pelvic organ prolapse (Bump and Norton, 1998).

Symptoms of pelvic floor dysfunction/ definitions

The symptom of urinary incontinence is defined as "complaint of involuntary loss of urine" with prevalence rates in the general population of women aged between 15 and 64 years varying between 32% and 64%. Most studies report prevalence rates between 25% and 45%. The most common symptom of female urinary incontinence is stress urinary incontinence which is defined as "complaint of involuntary loss of urine on effort or physical exertion or on sneezing and coughing." Urgency urinary incontinence is defined as "complaint of involuntary loss of urine associated with urgency" (typically leaking before reaching the toilet) and mixed urinary incontinence is a combination of stress and urgency incontinence. According to these definitions, it is easy to understand that stress urinary incontinence may unmask during physical activity.

Anal incontinence is defined as the involuntary loss of feces—solid or liquid (fecal incontinence) and involuntary loss of flatus. Anal and urinary incontinence often coexist, and prevalence rates of anal incontinence vary between 11% and 15% in the adult population.

Pelvic organ prolapse refers to loss of support for the uterus, bladder, colon, or rectum, leading to descent of one or more of these organs into the vagina. Pelvic organ prolapse quantification examination defines prolapse by measuring the descent of specific segments of the reproductive tract during valsalva strain relative to the hymen:

Stage 0: No prolapse is demonstrated.

Stage I: Most distal portion of the prolapse is more than 1 cm above the level of the hymen.

Stage II: Most distal portion of the prolapse is 1 cm or less proximal to or distal to the plane of the hymen.

Stage III: The most distal portion of the prolapse is more than 1 cm below the plane of the hymen.

Stage IV: Complete eversion of the total length of the lower genital tract is demonstrated. The prevalence of anatomic prolapse is about 30%, whereas sysmptomatic prolapse (a sensation of a mass bulging into the vagina) is ranging betweeen 5% and 10%.

Well-established etiological factors for pelvic floor dysfunction include pregnancy and vaginal childbirth (instrumental deliveries increase the risk), older age, obesity, and gynecological surgery. Other factors are less clear, such as strenuous work or exercise, constipation with straining on stool, chronic coughing, or other conditions that increase abdominal pressure chronically.

Pelvic floor and strenuous physical activity

There are two hypotheses about the pelvic floor and strenuous exercise, going in totally opposite directions.

Hypothesis one: female athletes have strong pelvic floor muscles

The rationale behind this hypothesis is that any physical activity that increases intra-abdominal pressure will lead to a simultaneous co-contraction or precontraction of the PFM, thereby giving a training stimulus to the muscles. Based on this assumption, general physical activity would prevent and treat stress urinary incontinence, but has also raised concern that elite athletes develop a stiff and rigid pelvic floor that may increase the risk of prolonged second stage of labor and lead to instrumental delivery. However, women leak during physical activity, and they report worse leakage during high-impact activities. To date, there is scant knowledge about elite athletes and delivery outcomes, but there is no strong evidence that elite athletes have more difficult childbirth than their sedentary counterparts. To the author's knowledge, no sport activities involve a direct voluntary contraction of the PFM, and it is unlikely that the athletes would be aware of the pelvic floor during activity. Furthermore, many women do not demonstrate an effective simultaneous or precontraction of the PFM during increased abdominal pressure, this being the reason for why they leak. In nulliparous women, stress urinary incontinence may be due to genetically weak connective tissue, location of the PFM at a lower, caudal position inside the pelvis, lower total number of muscle fibers (especially fast-twitch fibers), or untrained muscles in those leaking.

To date, there is little knowledge about PFM function in elite athletes. Our group measured PFM function in sport and physical education students with and without urinary incontinence and did not find any difference in PFM strength. The increase in PFM pressure during a voluntary contraction was 16.2 cmH$_2$O (SD 8.7) in the group with stress urinary incontinence and 14.3 cmH$_2$O (SD 8.2) in the continent group. However, this study was limited by its small sample size, and no strong conclusion can be drawn.

Hypothesis two: female athletes may overload, stretch, and weaken the pelvic floor

Heavy lifting and strenuous work have been listed as risk factors for the development of pelvic organ prolapse and stress urinary incontinence. It has been suggested that the cardinal and uterosacral ligaments, PFM, and the connective tissue of the perineum might be damaged chronically because of repeatedly increase in abdominal pressure due to hard manual work and chronic cough. To date, there are still few data to support the hypothesis. In a study of Danish nursing assistants, it was found that they were 1.6 times more likely to undergo surgery for genital prolapse and incontinence than women in the general population. However, the study did not control for parity. Hence, it is difficult to conclude whether heavy lifting is an etiological factor.

In the United States Air Force female crew, 26% of women capable of sustaining up to 9 G reported urinary incontinence. However, more women had incontinence off duty than while flying, and it was concluded that flying high-performance military aircraft did not affect the rate of incontinence. Nine of 420 nulliparous female soldiers entering the airborne infantry training program developed severe incontinence. Hence, most women were not negatively affected by this high-impact activity.

The maximum vertical ground reaction forces during different sport activities have been reported to be 3–4 times body weight for running, 5–12 times for jumping, 9 times for landing from front somersault, 14 times for landing after double back somersault, 16 times during landing in long jumps, and 9 times body weight in the lead foot in javelin throwing. Thus, one would anticipate that the pelvic floor of athletes needs to be much stronger than in the normal population to counteract these forces. Several studies have found that coughing and valsalva (as in defecation) increase intra-abdominal pressure to a significantly higher degree than different daily movements and exercises. Many exercises including abdominal exercise did not increase the intra-abdominal pressure more than rising up from a chair. In a recent study, PFM strength was compared in 10 handball, 10 volleyball, and 10 basketball players, as well as a nonexercising control group, and weaker muscles were found in the volleyball and basketball players compared with the controls. Lower strength correlated with increased symptoms of urinary incontinence.

Our group found that one bout of 90 minutes of strenuous exercise significantly reduced maximum voluntary contraction of the PFMs in nulliparous women with stress urinary incontinence with 17%. No change was seen in muscle endurance or vaginal resting pressure, and we do not know how long the reduced strength was present or whether this improved strength later on. In another study, 10 elite athletes were compared with 10 age-matched controls using MRI and found that there was no difference in the area of the levator hiatus, but there was a 20% higher cross-sectional area of the levator ani muscle in the athletes. The authors speculated whether this may give longer second stage of labor. In a follow-up study, they assessed 24 nulliparous elite athletes (with at least 5 years at national or international standard involving high-impact activity sports) and compared them with age- and body mass index (BMI)-matched controls. They confirmed the higher muscle diameter of the PFMs, but found larger levator hiatus area and more descent of the bladder in the athletes versus the controls during valsalva. There was no difference in hiatal area at rest or during PFM contraction. A larger levator hiatus area may facilitate normal vaginal birth and contradicts the first hypothesis. More research is needed in this important area of female elite athletes and the pelvic floor.

Although the prevalence of urinary incontinence is high, many athletes do not leak during strenuous activities and high increases in intra-abdominal pressure. However, from a theoretical understanding of functional anatomy and biomechanics, it is likely that heavy lifting and strenuous activity may promote these conditions in women already at risk (e.g., those with benign hypermobility joint syndrome or a large levator hiatus area may be predisposed for pelvic floor dysfunction). Physical activity may unmask and exaggerate the condition. Two studies investigated former elite athletes 15–20 years after their sport career and did not find any difference in urinary incontinence between those who had participated in low- versus high-impact activities or between former athletes and controls, respectively. However, women experiencing urinary incontinence at an early stage were more likely to report urinary incontinence later in life. Hence, it is important to start prevention and early treatment of the condition. There is a need for further studies to understand the influence of different exercises and strenuous physical activity on the pelvic floor.

Prevalence of pelvic floor dysfunction in female elite athletes

Urinary incontinence

An overview of published studies on prevalence of urinary incontinence in elite athletes is shown in Table 8.1. There is a high prevalence of symptoms of both stress and urgency urinary incontinence in young nulliparous, as well as parous elite athletes. Two studies compared the prevalence of incontinence in elite athletes with that of age-matched controls. Equal prevalences of stress and urgency urinary incontinence were found in athletes and controls. However, the prevalence of leakage during physical activities was significantly higher in the elite athletes. One study found a significantly higher prevalence in elite athletes compared with both physically active and sedentary controls.

As seen from Table 8.1, the question on incontinence was posed in different ways (e.g., leakage during past week or last 6 months) and was not always well described. One research group also measured urinary leakage in the elite trampolinists who reported the leakage to be a problem during trampoline training. The leakage was verified in all participants with a mean leakage of 28 g (range 9–56) in a 15-minute test on the trampoline. PFM function was measured in a subgroup of 10 women. They were all classified as having strong voluntary contractions by vaginal palpation, pointing out that timing of the automatic response by the PFM has not been adequate. Urinary incontinence has been reported to occur more frequently during the learning phase of new movements and during the last part of the training sessions and competitions.

There is limited knowledge about associated factors with stress urinary incontinence in athletes. In a study of college athletes, no significant association between incontinence and amenorrhea, weight, hormonal therapy or duration of athletic activity was found. In a study of former Olympians, they found that among factors such as age, body mass index (BMI), parity, Olympic sport group, and incontinence during Olympic sport 20 years ago, only current BMI was significantly associated with regular stress or urgency urinary incontinence symptoms. One study reported that significantly more elite athletes with eating disorders had symptoms of both stress and urgency urinary incontinence, and one study found that incontinent trampolinists were significantly older (16 vs. 13 years), had been training longer and more frequently, and were less able to interrupt the urine flow stream by voluntarily contracting the PFM than the nonleaking group.

A high proportion of athletes report that the leakage is embarrassing, affects their sport performance, or is a social or hygienic problem. One study reported that even small quantities of urine loss caused embarrassment, and 84% of the athletes had never spoken to anyone about the condition. One can imagine that urinary incontinence is more of a problem in sports with focus on the individual and where leakage is visible, for example, esthetic sports. In some sports such as gymnastics, lack of focus and concentration during sport can be dangerous.

Anal incontinence

There is sparse knowledge about anal incontinence during physical activity. Anecdotally, both male and female athletes may pass wind and feces during heavy lifting. One recent study included female students, age 18–40, years from sport, physiotherapy, and nursing in southern France. They found a statistically significant higher prevalence of anal incontinence in those performing intensive sport, defined as training more than 8 hours per week compared with all other subjects (14.8% vs. 4.9%, respectively, $p = 0.001$). Anal incontinence was mainly represented by loss of flatus (84%). As for urinary incontinence, anal incontinence is probably more of a problem in sports where this can be seen or heard.

Table 8.1 Prevalence of urinary incontinence in female elite athletes

	Design	Population/sample	Response rate	Question	Results
Nygaard et al. 1994	Cross-sectional Postal survey	All women participating in competitive varsity athletics at a large state university in USA (n = 156) Mean age 19.9 years ± 3.3 (SD) Nulliparous	92%	Have you ever experienced unanticipated urinary leakage during participation in your sport, coughing, sneezing, heavy lifting, walking to the bathroom, sleeping, and upon hearing the sound of running water?	28% reported at least one episode of urinary incontinence while practicing or competing in their sport Gymnastics: 67% Tennis: 50% Basketball: 44% Field hockey: 32% Track: 26% Volleyball: 9% Swimming: 6% Softball: 6% Golf: 0% 42% experienced urine loss during daily activities 38% felt embarrassed
Nygaard 1997	Retrospective and cross-sectional Postal survey	Former American female Olympians (between 1960 and 1976) participating in gymnastics and track and field compared with swimmers (n = 207) Mean age: 44.3 years (range 30–63) Mean number of years since beginning training: 30	51.2%	Do you now/did you while being Olympian participant experience urinary leakage related to feeling of urgency, or related to activity, coughing, or sneezing	While Olympians: Swimming: 4.5% Gymnastics/track and field: 35.0% (p<0.005) Now: Swimming: 50% Gymnastics/track and field: 41% (ns)
Bø and Borgen (2001)	Cross-sectional, case-control Postal questionnaire	All female elite athletes on national team or recruiting squad in Norway (n = 660) and age-matched controls (n = 765) Age: 15–39 years Parity: 5% in elite athletes, 33% in controls	Athletes: 87% Controls: 75%	Do you currently leak urine during coughing, sneezing and laughter, physical activity (running and jumping, abrupt movements, and lifting) or with urge to void (problems in reaching the toilet without leaking?	Stress urinary continence (SUI) Athletes: 41% Controls: 39% Range between sports: 37.5–52.2% Urge: Athletes: 16% Controls: 19% Range between sports: 10–27.5% Social/hygienic problem: Athletes: 15% Controls: 16.4% Moderate/severe problem: Athletes/controls: 5%

Study	Design	Participants	Prevalence	Question	Results
Thyssen et al. 2002	Cross-sectional Postal survey	Eight Danish sport clubs (including ballet) competing at national level (n = 397) Mean age: 22.8 years (range 14–51) 8.6% were parous	73.7%	Do you experience urine loss while participating in your sport or in daily life?	51.9% experienced urine loss during sport or in daily life. 43% while participating in their sport: Gymnastics: 56% Ballet: 43% Aerobics: 40% Badminton: 31% Volleyball: 30% Athletics: 25% Handball: 21% Basketball: 17%
Eliasson et al. 2002	Cross-sectional Postal survey Clinical assessment: pad test during trampoline training (n = 18), measurement of PFM strength (n = 10)	All 35 female Swedish trampolinists at national level between 1993 and 1996 Mean age 15 (range 12–22) Nulliparous	100% on survey 51.4% on pad test 28.6% on strength measurement	Do you leak urine during trampoline training/competition/daily life?	80% reported to leak urine during trampoline training/competition and sport. None leaked during coughing, sneezing, or laughing 51.4% reported the leakage to be embarrassing Mean leakage on pad testing: 28 grams (range 9–56)
Caylet et al. 2006	Cross-sectional study comparing athletes and controls Postal survey	157 elite athletes at highest national level in Nimes, France, compared with random sample of 426 controls Age: 18–35 years Nulliparous	55.6% of athletes and 70% of controls	Do you leak urine during coughing, sneezing, laughing, sudden change in position, cold exposure, hand washing, loud noises, anxiety, or physical activity (first or second part of training or competition? Rating as slight or marked and frequency as daily, weekly, or monthly. Embarrassment on visual analog scale (VAS) scale	Athletes: 28% Physically active controls and sedentary controls: 9.8% Most reported only a few episodes per month. 8% several episodes per day
Vitton et al. 2011	Cross-sectional study Postal questionnaire comparing high-level sport (>8 hours per week) and nonintensive sport (all other groups) participants	393 of 750 eligible women age 18–40, from Sport University, School of Physiotherapy and School of Nursing in Marseille, France Nulliparous	52.4%	Did you have an accidental anal leakage of solid, liquid, mucus, or gas at least once in the last 6 months? If yes: type of protection worn, leakage composition, leakage duration, and frequency Did you have an accidental urinary leakage at least once during the last 6 months? If yes: type of protection worn, leakage duration, and frequency	Anal incontinence: 14.8% in intensive sport (IS) versus 4.9% in nonintensive sport (NIS) ($p<0.01$) Anal incontinence was mainly flatus: 84% Urinary incontinence: 33.1% versus 18.3% ($p<0.01$)

Pelvic organ prolapse

Although there are anecdotal reports of pelvic organ prolapse in young, nulliparous marathon runners and weight lifters, there are few studies on pelvic organ prolapse in exercising women. In a study comparing nulliparous women before and after 6 weeks of summer military training, it was found that women attending paratrooper training were significantly more likely to have stage II prolapse. They were also significantly more likely to have worsening in their pelvic support regardless of initial prolapse stage.

Prevention of pelvic floor dysfunction

There are no studies applying PFMT for primary prevention of urinary incontinence, anal incontinence, or pelvic organ prolapse in the general female population or in elite athletes. Theoretically, one could argue that strengthening the PFM by specific training would have the potential to prevent stress urinary incontinence, anal incontinence, and pelvic organ prolapse. Strength training of the PFM has shown to increase the thickness of the muscles, reduce muscle length, reduce the levator hiatus area, and lift the levator plate to a more cranial level inside the pelvis in women with pelvic organ prolapse. If the pelvic floor possesses a certain "stiffness," it is likely that the muscles could counteract the increases in intra-abdominal pressures occurring during physical exertion.

Preventive devices and absorbing products

Devices that involve external urinary collection, intravaginal support of the bladder neck, or blockage of urinary leakage by occlusion are available, and some have shown to be effective in preventing leakage during physical activity. A vaginal tampon can be such a simple device. In a Danish study, six women with SUI demonstrated total dryness when using a vaginal device during 30 minutes of aerobics. This was supported by a recent study in 34 Australian women. However, in the latter study, only 47% of the participants reported high acceptability for tampon use. For smaller leakage, specially designed protecting pads can be used during training and competition.

Treatment of pelvic floor dysfunction in elite athletes

Stress urinary incontinence

Stress urinary incontinence can be treated with bladder training, PFMT with or without resistance devices, vaginal cones or biofeedback, electrical stimulation, drug therapy, or surgery. One would assume that the elite athletes would respond in the same way to treatment as other women do. However, given the high impact on their pelvic floor, they may need stronger PFM than nonathletes. To date, there are methodological problems assessing PFM, bladder, and urethral function during physical activity.

Surgery

Elite athletes are mostly young and nulliparous, and it is therefore recommended that PFMT should be the first choice of treatment and is always tried before surgery. The leakage in athletes seems to be related to strenuous high-impact activity, and elite athletes do not seem to have more urinary incontinence than others later in life when the activity is reduced. Therefore, surgery seems inappropriate in young elite athletes.

Bladder training

Anecdotally, most elite athletes empty their bladder before practice and competition, which was also reported to be common in young nulliparous women attending gyms. Therefore, it is unlikely that any of them would exercise with a high bladder volume. However, as in the rest of the population, elite athletes may have a nonoptimal toilet behavior, and the use of frequency–volume chart and bladder training regimens may be an important first step to become aware of toilet habits and try to make them more optimal.

Estrogen

The role of estrogen in incidence, prevalence, and treatment of stress urinary incontinence is controversial. Two meta-analyses of the effect have concluded that there is no change in urine loss after estrogen replacement therapy. Estrogen given alone therefore does not seem to be an effective treatment for stress urinary incontinence. A higher prevalence of eating disorders has been found in athletes compared with nonathletes, and these athletes may be low in estrogen. Amenorrheic elite athletes would be on estrogen replacement therapy because of the risk of osteoporosis. Estrogen may have adverse effects such as a higher risk of coronary heart disease and some cancer forms.

Pelvic floor muscle training

Based on systematic reviews and meta-analysis of randomized controlled trials, it has been stated that conservative treatments with lifestyle interventions and PFMT should be first-line treatment for stress and mixed urinary incontinence. Cochrane reviews conclude that PFMT is an effective treatment for adult women and consistently better than no treatment or placebo treatments. Subjective cure and improvement rates after PFMT for stress urinary or mixed incontinence reported in randomized controlled trials to be up to 70%. Cure rates, defined as ≤2 g of leakage on pad tests, vary between 44 and 70% in stress urinary incontinence. Supervised training shows better results than unsupervised training. Adverse effects have only been reported in one study. One woman out of 54 reported pain with PFM contractions; three had an uncomfortable feeling during exercise; and two felt that they did not want to be continually occupied with the problem.

No randomized controlled trials on the effect of PFMT on urinary incontinence have been conducted in elite athletes. In one study, 39 female soldiers, mean age 28.5 years (SD 7.2), with exercise-induced urinary incontinence were randomized to PFMT with or without biofeedback. All improved subjectively and showed normal readings on urodynamic assessment after treatment. Only eight subjects desired further treatment after 8 weeks of training.

Two small case series on elite athletes and sport students have been published. One study reported total relief of reported symptoms and no leakage on pad testing after 3 months of a combination of electrical stimulation, PFMT with biofeedback, and vaginal cones. In another study it was reported that seven nulliparous sport students significantly improved PFM strength and reduced urinary incontinence score, frequency and amount of leakage after 8 weeks of training.

Elite athletes are accustomed to regular training and are highly motivated for exercise. Adding three sets of 8–12 close to maximum contractions, 3–4 times a week of the PFM to their regular strength-training program does not seem to be a big task. However, there is no reason to believe that they are more able than the general population to perform a correct PFM contraction. Therefore, thorough instruction and assessment of ability to contract is mandatory. Because most elite athletes are nulliparous, there are no ruptures of ligaments, fascias, muscle fibers, or peripheral nerve damage. One would expect that the effect would be equal or even better in this specific group of women. On the other hand, the impact and increase in abdominal pressure that has to be counteracted by the PFM in athletes performing high-impact activities is much higher than what is required in the sedentary population. The pelvic floor therefore probably needs to be much stronger in elite athletes.

There are two different theoretical rationales for the effect of PFMT. A voluntary contraction of the PFM before and during cough reduced leakage by 98 and 73% during a medium and deep cough, respectively. Kegel first described the PFMT method in 1948 as "tightening" of the pelvic floor. The rationale behind a strength-training regimen is to increase muscle tension and cross-sectional area and increase stiffness of connective tissue, thereby lifting the pelvic floor into a higher pelvic position and reduce the levator hiatus area. This effect has been verified in a randomized controlled trial.

It is unlikely that continent elite athletes or participants in fitness activities think about the

PFM or precontract them voluntarily. A contraction of the PFM most likely occurs automatically and simultaneously or even before the impact or abdominal pressure increase. It seems impossible to voluntarily precontract the PFM before and during every increase in abdominal pressure while participating in sport and leisure activities. The aim of the training program therefore would be to build up the PFM to a firm structural base where such contractions occur automatically.

Most likely, very few, if any, athletes have learned about the PFM, and one could assume that none have tried to train them systematically. The potential for improvement in function and strength is therefore huge. PFMT has proved to be effective when conducted intensively and with a close follow-up in the general population. It is a functional and physiological noninvasive treatment with no known serious adverse effects, and it is cost-effective compared with other treatment modalities. However, there is a need for high-quality randomized controlled trial (RCTs) to evaluate the effect of PFM strength training in female elite athletes.

Prevention and treatment of anal incontinence

There are no randomized controlled trials on the effect of surgical or conservative management of anal incontinence in the nulliparous population or in athletes. The results of PFMT in women with perineal tears after childbirth and in women with anal incontinence following childbirth are inconsistent and inconclusive. There is some evidence that women performing antenatal PFMT are less likely to have anal incontinence postpartum.

Prevention and treatment of pelvic organ prolapse

No randomized controlled trials, or studies using other designs, have been found to evaluate the effect of lifestyle interventions or PFMT on pelvic organ prolapse in primary prevention, that is, to stop prolapse from developing. To date, eight randomized controlled trials have evaluated the effect of PFMT to treat anatomical prolapse or symptoms. Typically, most randomized controlled trials

compared PFMT plus lifestyle intervention, against lifestyle interventions alone. Lifestyle intervention included the use of precontraction of the PFM before and during increase in intra-abdominal pressure, "the Knack" and advice to avoid pushing down during defecation or general lifestyle advice. None have compared the effect of these lifestyle interventions with untreated controls, and there is no report of adherence to these protocols. Hence, the effect of lifestyle interventions on pelvic organ prolapse is still unknown. In one randomized controlled trial, there was no effect of advice to use the Knack on PFM morphology.

The results of the randomized controlled trials are all in favor of PFMT to be effective in treating pelvic organ prolapse, demonstrating statistically significant improvement in symptoms and/or prolapse stage. Typically, anatomical position of the prolapse is improved by one stage.

Conclusion

The prevalence of urinary incontinence and especially stress urinary incontinence among young, nulliparous elite athletes is high. The highest prevalence rates were found in those involved in high-impact activities such as trampolining, gymnastics, track and field, and ball games. Anal incontinence in the form of loss of flatus is also common. Both urinary and anal incontinence is perceived as embarrassing, and it may influence performance especially in sports where incontinence is visible or hearable. There is scant knowledge about the prevalence of pelvic organ prolapse in female athletes. There are no randomized controlled trials on the effect of prevention or treatment of incontinence or pelvic organ prolapse in female elite athletes. There is strong evidence that PFMT is effective in the treatment of stress and mixed urinary incontinence and pelvic organ prolapse in the general population, it has no adverse effects and is recommended as first-line treatment in the adult female population. There is a need for more basic research on PFM function during physical activity, exercise as an etiological factor for pelvic floor dysfunction, and the effect of PFMT in female elite athletes.

Recommendations for effective PFMT for elite athletes

• Be sure that correct contraction is performed before starting the program. This is best assessed by a trained women's health/pelvic floor physiotherapist.
• Self-test of correct PFM contraction can be done by trying to stop the dribbling at the end of voiding or placing one hand on the perineum. If performed correctly, the woman will feel the lift away from the hand.
• Use positions with legs apart to avoid too much co-contraction of other muscle groups.
• Perform 8–12 close to maximum contraction for 6–8 seconds, three sets per day.
• Make progression by contracting harder and increase the holding period without increasing the intra-abdominal pressure.
• Avoid straining on toilet.
• Precontract the PFM before and during coughing and sneezing.

References

Bø K and Borgen JS. (2001) Prevalence of stress and urge urinary incontinence in elite athletes and controls. *Med Sci Sports Exerc*, 33, 1797–1802.

Bump R and Norton P. (1998) Epidemiology and natural history of pelvic floor dysfunction. *Obstet Gyn Clin N Am*, 25(4), 723–746.

Caylet N, Fabbro-Peray P, Mares P, Dauzat M, Prat-Pradal D, and Corcos J. (2006) Prevalence and occurrence of stress urinary incontinence in elite women athletes. *Can J Urol*, 13(4), 3174–3179.

Eliasson K, Larsson T, and Mattson E. (2002) Prevalence of stress incontinence in nulliparous elite trampolinists. *Scand J Med Sci Sports*, 12, 106–110.

Nygaard I, Thompson FL, Svengalis SL, et al. (1994) Urinary incontinence in elite nulliparous athletes. *Obstet Gynecol*, 84, 183–187.

Nygaard IE. (1997) Does prolonged high-impact activity contribute to later urinary incontinence? A retrospective cohort study of female Olympians. *Obst Gynecol*, 90, 718–722.

Thyssen HH, Clevin L, Olesen S et al. (2002) Urinary incontinence in elite female athletes and dancers. *Int Urogynecology J Pelvic Floor Dysfunct*, 13, 15–17.

Vitton V, Baumstarck-Barrau K, Brardjanian S. Caballe I, Bouvier M, and Grimaud JC. (2011) Impact of high-level sport practice on anal incontinence in a healthy young female population. *J Women's Health*, 20(5), 757–763.

Recommended reading

Borin LCMS, Nunes FR, and Guirro ECOG. (2013) Assessment of pelvic floor muscle pressure in female athletes. *Physical Med Rehab*, 5, 189–193.

Brækken IH, Majida M, Engh ME, and Bø K. (2010) Morphological changes after pelvic floor muscle training measured by 3-dimensional ultrasonography: a randomized controlled trial. *Obstet Gynecol*, 115(2), 317–324.

Bø K. (2004) Urinary incontinence, pelvic floor dysfunction, exercise and sport. *Sport Med*, 34(7), 451–464.

Bø K and Sundgot-Borgen J. (2010) Are former female elite athletes more likely to experience urinary incontinence later in life than non-athletes? *Scand J Med Sci Sports*, 20, 100–104.

Hay J. (1993) Citius, altius, longius (faster, higher, longer): the biomechanics of jumping for distance. *J Biomech*, 26(1), 7–21.

Haylen BT, de Ridder D, Freeman RM, et al. (2010) An International Urogynecological Association (IUGA)/ International Continence Society (ICS) joint report on the terminology for female pelvic floor dysfunction. *Int Urogynecol J Pelvic Floor Dysfunct*, 21, 5–26.

Milsom I, Altman D, Cartwright R, et al. (2013) Epidemiology of urinary incontinence (UI) and other lower urinary tract symptoms (LUTS), pelvic organ prolapse (POP) and anal incontinence. In: P Abrams L Cardozo A Khoury and A Wein (eds), *4th International Consultation on Urinary Incontinence* (5th edn, pp. 15–107). Health Publication Ltd: Plymbridge Committee 1.

Moore K, Dumoulin C, Bradley C, et al. (2013) Adult conservative management. In: P Abrams L Cardozo S Khouy and A Wein (eds), *5th International Consultation on Urinary Incontinence* (5th edn, pp. 1101–1227). Health Publication Ltd: Plymbridge Committee 12.

Chapter 9
Female athlete triad

Marci Goolsby

Women's Sports Medicine Center, Hospital for Special Surgery New York, NY, USA

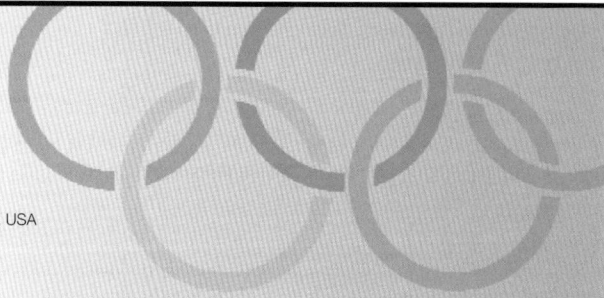

Introduction

The female athlete triad ("Triad") refers to the relationship between three components: energy availability, menstrual function, and bone health. The Triad was first described in the early 1990s, and the American College of Sports Medicine (ACSM) published the first position stand on the Triad in 1997 with a revised version published in 2007. The revised version focused on the spectrum of disease seen, rather than only the diagnoses seen at the extreme end of pathology: amenorrhea (lack of menses), low energy availability with or without disordered eating, and osteoporosis. Recognizing athletes at risk who may not yet demonstrate the more severe disease of this spectrum is important for early intervention. There are a myriad of negative consequences of the Triad that are preventable. Thus, there has been a lot of focus on education of athletes, coaches, health care providers and others. Adolescence and young adulthood is a critical time in bone and reproductive health, making the early identification of the Triad important in order to minimize the short-term and long-term consequences.

Components and consequences

The Triad describes three components and their interrelationship (see Figure 9.1). These three components exist along a spectrum from healthy energy balance to low energy availability with or without disordered eating, normal menstrual function to amenorrhea, and good bone health to osteoporosis. Athletes may demonstrate one or more of these three components and early diagnosis and intervention are critical to preventing further progression of disease. Challenges exist in studies of prevalence due to variable definitions and techniques for studying the components, often relying on inaccurate assessment tools. Despite these challenges, there is evidence for an increased incidence of the Triad components among exercising women, particularly those involved in leanness sports such as endurance (i.e., distance running), weight class (i.e., wrestling), and aesthetic sports (i.e., figure skating).

Energy availability

Energy availability refers to the balance between dietary calorie intake and exercise energy expenditure. When the calories burned with exercise exceed the calories from nutrition intake, this is referred to as low energy availability. Often, this occurs with disordered eating where the athlete practices unhealthy eating habits such as restricting overall calorie intake or avoiding certain foods

The Female Athlete, First Edition. Edited by Margo L. Mountjoy.
© 2015 International Olympic Committee. Published 2015 by John Wiley & Sons, Inc.

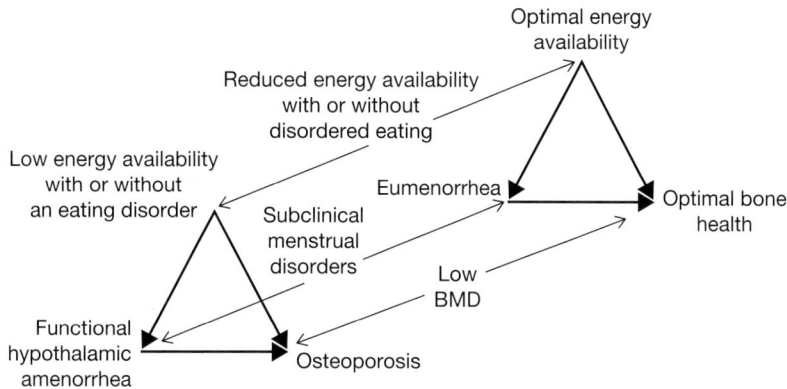

Figure 9.1 Female athlete triad. The spectrums of energy availability, menstrual function, and bone mineral density along which female athletes are distributed (narrow arrows). An athlete's condition moves along each spectrum at a different rate, in one direction or the other, according to her diet and exercise habits. Energy availability, defined as dietary energy intake minus exercise energy expenditure, affects BMD both directly via metabolic hormones and indirectly via effects on menstrual function and thereby estrogen (thick arrows). Reprinted with permission from Nattiv et al. (2007).

but without meeting the clinical criteria for the diagnosis of an eating disorder. Clinical eating disorders can also occur such as anorexia nervosa, bulimia nervosa, and eating disorder not otherwise specified. Recognition of the eating disorder signs is particularly important in the Olympic athletes as elite athletes are three times more likely to have an eating disorder than the general population (Sundgot-Borgen and Torstveit, 2004). Excessive exercise is often a contributing factor as well, particularly in elite athletes, and the athlete may be exercising more than is appropriate for their training in order to lose weight. The imbalance can also be accidental in the case of an athlete who has an increased or overall strenuous training without appropriate adjustment of her nutrition. Low energy availability in turn disrupts the hormonal pathways, which is manifested clinically as menstrual dysfunction, or irregular periods. Inadequate nutrition can have detrimental effects on performance through associated fatigue, dehydration, vitamin deficiencies, anemia, higher risk of injury, depression, and poor recovery.

Menstrual function

The hypothalamic–pituitary–gonadal hormone axis is disrupted by the low energy availability and can lead to a number of reproductive disturbances, most often seen clinically as oligomenorrhea and amenorrhea. Oligomenorrhea refers to prolonged time between menses (more than 35 days). Primary amenorrhea is lack of onset of menstruation (menarche) by age 15 years. Secondary amenorrhea refers to lack of menses for more than 3 months after menarche has occurred. Specifically, the type of amenorrhea seen in the Triad is functional hypothalamic amenorrhea, describing the disruption of the hormone axis. The incidence of functional hypothalamic amenorrhea varies by sport but has been reported as high as 65% in distance runners (Dusek, 2001). Other menstrual dysfunction can occur that is not as clinically apparent such as anovulatory cycles and luteal phase dysfunction; therefore, normal menses does not always mean low energy availability is not present. The consequences of disrupted hormonal function include both short- and long-term effects on fertility and bone health.

Bone health

Both nutritional deficits and hormonal disruption can have a negative impact on bone health, leading to an increased risk of stress fractures as well as the risk of developing early osteoporosis. Research has shown a dose–response effect of Triad risk factors on low bone mineral density (BMD) incidence

(Gibbs *et al.*, 2013). A woman reaches her maximum bone health potential in young adulthood, thus making this a critical time for adequate nutrition and avoidance of negative factors. With prolonged nutritional and menstrual disturbances, this negative impact on bone may not be fully reversible. Delayed menarche, history of oligomenorrhea or amenorrhea, and low BMD have all been associated with an increased risk of stress injuries to the bone. These can significantly impact an athlete's career due to missed training and competition. The impact of osteoporosis on morbidity and mortality in the older population has been well described with half of all women suffering an osteoporosis-related fracture over the age of 50 and a quarter of seniors who break their hip will die within 1 year.

Screening and risk factors

Unlike many ailments female athletes may suffer from, the Triad may not be obvious. It is particularly important then for doctors, athletic trainers, coaches, others involved in care of athletes, and the athletes themselves to be aware of the risk factors. Early recognition may prevent some of the negative consequences on injury risk, performance, reproductive health, mental well-being, and the long-term risk of osteoporosis. One of the biggest risk factors for developing the Triad is the type of sport. The Triad is more commonly seen in sports that emphasize leanness such as endurance, weight class, and aesthetic sports where appearance may play a role in competition. However, the Triad has been seen in many sports, so all female athletes should be screened for the risk factors and components. There are a number of risk factors that have been identified for eating disorders such as societal pressure, dieting, "perfectionist" personality, and family history of eating disorder. A comment from a coach, parent, or peer can also precipitate disordered eating behaviors, particularly if there are positive responses to initial weight loss that perpetuate the disorder. In athletes, specifically, there is often the misconception that losing weight or body fat will improve performance. Questions related to the Triad components should

be a part of every screening evaluation. Ideally, screening should begin as young as possible in athletes. The IOC proposes a history form for use in periodic health evaluations of elite athletes that can be found in the Appendix. In summary, athletes should be asked about the following:

1 injury history, particularly stress fractures;
2 menstrual history, both current and past; and
3 nutrition and weight history, including eating disorder diagnoses, highest and lowest recent weight, and thoughts/feelings toward their nutrition/weight.

The number, location, and severity (time missed) of stress fractures is important to ask. A history of traumatic fractures should also be part of injury history. In menstrual history, age of menarche, history of menstrual pattern, and recent menstrual pattern are all important as is asking about medications that may impact menses such as contraceptive pills, patches, or ring and medroxyprogesterone acetate injections (Depo-Provera). There are a number of screening tools available for identifying disordered eating habits with more detail that can be incorporated. Table 9.1 shows a series of questions that correlated eating habits with low BMD. A positive response to any of these questions should prompt further questions about the other components and risk factors and may need a separate detailed visit with a dietitian and/or mental health provider. A coach or teammate can help by notifying someone if they see the athlete engaging in unusual or unhealthy dietary habits such as eating small portion sizes, not eating in front of others, dieting, playing with her food, rapid weight loss, extra workouts beyond what the team or coach has advised, and/or frequent trips to the restroom after eating. There are also comments the athlete may make in reference to her weight, appearance, or eating that may be of concern. These concerns can be brought to others' attention so that the team of caretakers can get further information from the athlete. On physical examination, the physician should evaluate for signs of an eating disorder such as tooth enamel erosions, parotid gland swelling, calluses on the knuckles (Russell's sign), lanugo (fine body hair), as well as low BMI, weight change, significant bradycardia, orthostatic hypotension, and general thin appearance. If any components

Table 9.1 Dietary Restraint Questions (EDE-Q) correlated with low BMD in high school

Endurance runners

1. Have you been consciously trying to restrict the amount of food you eat to influence your shape or weight?
2. Have you gone for long periods of time (8 hours or more) without eating anything in order to influence your shape or weight?
3. Have you attempted to avoid eating any foods that you like in order to influence your shape or weight?
4. Have you attempted to follow definite rules regarding your eating in order to influence your shape or weight, for example a calorie limit, a set amount of food, or rules about what or when you should eat?
5. Have you had a definite desire for your stomach to feel empty?

Source: Reprinted with permission from IOC Consensus Statement on Periodic Health Evaluation of the Elite Athlete (2009).

or risk factors are identified in the screening process, it is important to follow up with a more comprehensive visit and involve other members of the team as indicated.

Diagnosis and further testing

Once a component or risk factor is identified, it is important to have a multidisciplinary team to aid in the diagnosis. For example, involving a registered dietitian can be critical to obtain a more comprehensive evaluation of dietary habits and assist in diagnosing low energy availability and/or disordered eating/eating disorder. Accurately measuring energy availability can be challenging in a clinical setting and requires information about exercise energy expenditure, total dietary caloric intake, and fat-free body mass, which requires measurement of body weight and body fat composition. There are many ways these assessments can be done, and it is best to involve a registered dietitian. Much of the information is self-reported by the athlete and can be challenging due to recall accuracy and even exaggeration of intake and/or minimizing exercise expenditure. Dietary intake can be evaluated with a diet log, ideally done over multiple days during a training period. Tools for measuring exercise expenditure are available including accelerometers and heart rate monitors but there

are other ways to estimate exercise energy expenditure including the 2011 Compendium of Physical Activities where exercise expenditure = activity MET × weight × hours of activity (Ainsworth *et al.*, 2011). Body fat composition can be measured using Dual-energy X-ray Absorptiometry (DXA), skin fold measurements, air displacement plethysmography, and bioelectrical impedance, depending on what is available. Energy availability can be calculated as energy intake (in kilocalories) minus exercise energy expenditure (in kilocalories) divided by fat-free mass (in kilograms). An online calculator is also available at www.femaleathletetriad.org/calculators.

A sports psychologist or other mental health care professional should visit with the athlete and assist in their diagnosis and treatment if disordered eating or an eating disorder is identified.

A DXA to evaluate BMD should be considered for those athletes with:

- a high-risk stress fracture (i.e., femoral neck, sacrum, pelvis);
- recurrent low-trauma fractures or recurrent stress injuries;
- diagnosis of an eating disorder or prolonged disordered eating; or
- prolonged menstrual dysfunction (less than six periods in the last 12 months).

The ACSM position stand of 2007 advised the diagnosis of osteoporosis in premenopausal athletes require both BMD Z-score ≤–2.0 and secondary clinical risk factors such as hypoestrogenism, stress fractures, and a history of nutritional deficiencies. With the above risk factors and a Z-score between –1.0 and –2.0, it is considered low BMD.

If the athlete has had menstrual dysfunction, recurrent stress injuries, and/or low BMD, further blood and urine testing may be indicated to evaluate for other causes. Before determining the athlete has functional hypothalamic amenorrhea, other causes of amenorrhea should be excluded. For secondary amenorrhea, this may include urine beta hCG (rule out pregnancy), prolactin (rule out prolactinoma), thyroid stimulating hormone (rule out thyroid disease), FSH (rule out premature ovarian failure), and, if there is concern for polycystic ovarian syndrome, testosterone and DHEA-sulfate. An estradiol level and/or progesterone challenge test can confirm hypoestrogenism. For primary amenorrhea, pelvic ultrasound and karyotype testing may also be indicated. In the setting of recurrent bone stress injuries, other causes of metabolic bone disease may need to be considered and vitamin D, metabolic panel, thyroid studies, parathyroid hormone, 24-hour urine calcium, and markers of bone turnover may be indicated. Once the diagnosis of the Triad is made and further evaluation is complete, the next step is to formulate a treatment plan and ensure safe participation in training.

Return to sport/clearance

Through the screening process, those athletes at risk can be identified. Using a multidisciplinary approach, the best plan for the athlete must be individualized and may need to include restriction of her participation. This is a necessary part to making sure the health and safety of the athlete is of highest priority. All of the risk factors need to be taken into account when considering the clearance of these athletes. Both the severity and number of risk factors are important. This is described in detail in the Consensus Statement on Treatment and Return to Play, which uses a cumulative risk score to provide guidelines on clearance and return to play. If the health care team decides the athlete is not safe for participation, it is helpful to have a contract with the athlete detailing compliance with visits and treatment plan and goals that must be accomplished before she is allowed to participate.

Treatment

Athletes who show signs of the Triad or risk factors should seek help immediately. Early recognition and treatment can prevent many of the negative consequences of the Triad. The focus of treatment should be on addressing the low energy availability. A sports dietitian can help formulate an individualized nutrition plan for the athlete and continued monitoring of compliance should be done with frequent visits. Often, particularly if disordered eating or an eating disorder is present, a mental health professional such as a sports psychologist and/or psychiatrist should be meeting with the athlete. Treatment may involve weight gain, an increase in caloric intake, and/or a decrease in exercise energy expenditure. Changes should be gradual and starting with a 20% increase in caloric intake is often a good beginning. As said though, the plan should be individualized. Total dietary and supplemental calcium of 1000–1300 mg daily and vitamin D of 600 IU daily (or adjusted if vitamin D not between 32 and 50 ng/mL) is recommended to maximize bone health. If the athlete has an injury such as a stress fracture, separate treatment for the injury will need to take place and may include modification of activities, modified weight bearing, and splinting or casting. Oral contraceptive pills have not been proven to improve BMD in amenorrheic subjects, but recent evidence in anorexic subjects shows transdermal estrogen with cyclic progesterone, though not effective for contraceptive, improves low BMD (Misra *et al.*, 2011) and may be an option in Triad athletes. Very rarely, medications are indicated in female athletes with osteoporosis and recurrent fractures who have failed all other treatments including hormone treatment. There is limited data and concern for the use of osteoporosis medications in women in their child-bearing years and thus should be used with great caution and only under the guidance of a specialist. The main focus of treatment should be on reversing the low energy availability through education and nutrition counseling.

Prevention

The best treatment plan for the Triad is to prevent it from happening in the first place. Education is the key to prevention, and the message needs to be received by athletes, trainers, coaches, administrators, and all involved in an athlete's career. There are online resources, such as the IOC's Triad awareness tool, Healthy Body Image (http://www.olympic.org/hbi), and the Web site of the Female Athlete Triad Coalition (www.femaleathletetriad.org) that can provide further education for coaches and athletes. All those involved in caring for athletes need to be working together to promote a healthy environment for competition and training. Focus should be on performance and positive body image and not on weight or body fat goals. Comments from coaches can have detrimental effects on how the athlete views her weight and body image. Coaches should not be involved in weight management of the athletes nor pressure the athletes to lose body fat or weight. If indicated, a dietitian can assist in a weight management assessment and plan. Female athletes at the Olympic level also have a social responsibility to ensure the positive body image message is passed on to the younger generations. The misconception that thinner is better needs to be finally put to rest, and, in its place, an image of good nutrition and healthy body image and weight can be promoted.

Conclusion

The Triad has negative consequences that may affect bone health, reproductive health, performance, and cause missed time from competition and training. It is critical that athletes and those who care for athletes be aware of the signs and symptoms of the Triad. If a risk factor or component is identified, further questioning should take place to assess for other factors. There should be a multidisciplinary team in place to ensure the best evaluation and treatment of these athletes and may include athletic trainers, physicians, mental health providers, and dietitians. Treatment should focus on education and nutrition counseling to address the underlying low energy availability. Multiple factors should be taken into consideration when determining clearance and return to play for these athletes and it may not be healthy for some athletes to continue training. In this situation, a contract with the athlete can clearly lay out goals for them to ensure compliance with treatment. The best treatment, however, is prevention. With further education, the focus on healthy body image and nutrition can keep our female athletes training in good health.

Appendix

Athlete PHE Form

MEDICAL HISTORY

Demographic

Personal Information

Last Name _____ First Name _____

Address: Street _____ City _____ Region _____

Post Code _____ Country _____

Preferred Language: _____

Birthdate: yyyy _____ /mm _____ /dd _____

Sex (M/F): _____

Phone: Home _____ Mobile _____

Emergency Contact 1: Name _____ Relationship _____ Phone _____

Emergency Contact 2: Name _____ Relationship _____ Phone _____

Health Care Insurance (company number): _____

Family Physician (name, phone number): _____

Background

The following questions ask for information regarding your personal background

What is your main sport? (sport, event/position): _____

Have you participated in other sports in the past (include those sports you have done competitively)? No❑   Yes ❑: _____

What is your ethnic origin?: _____

Do you have any religious convictions that could affect your medical treatment?	No ❑	Yes ❑

When was the last time you had a complete physical examination?: _____

Have you ever failed a pre-participation examination for sports, or has your doctor ever stopped you from participating in sports for any reason?	No ❑	Yes ❑

In total, how many days have you missed practice or competition in the past year because of injury or illness?: _____

Heart

Have you ever had any of the following heart or circulation related problems?:

Chest pain, discomfort, tighness or pressure with exercise?	No ❑	Yes ❑
Unexplained fainting or near fainting or passed out for no reason DURING or AFTER exercise?	No ❑	Yes ❑
Excessive or unexplained shortness of breath, lightheaded, or fatigue with exercise?	No ❑	Yes ❑
Do you get more tired or short of breath more quickly than your friends during exercise?	No ❑	Yes ❑
Does your heart race or skip beats (irregular beats) during exercise?	No ❑	Yes ❑
Heart murmur, high blood pressure, high cholesterol, heart infection or inflammation, rheumatic fever, heart valve problems, or any other heart related problem?	No ❑	Yes ❑
Have you ever had an unexplained seizure?	No ❑	Yes ❑
Any tests for your heart (for example, ECG or EKG, echocardiogram)?	No ❑	Yes ❑

Breathing

Have you ever had any of the following respiratory or breathing problems:

Do you have asthma?	No ❑	Yes ❑
Do you have any other symptoms of respiratory (lung) disease including, wheezing, cough, postnasal drip, hay fever, or repeated flu like illness?	No ❑	Yes ❑
Do you cough, wheeze or have more difficulty breathing than you should during or after exercise?	No ❑	Yes ❑
Have you ever used asthma medication (such as an inhaler)?	No ❑	Yes ❑
Have you ever had bronchitis, pneumonia, tuberculosis, cystic fibrosis or other respiratory or other breathing problem?	No ❑	Yes ❑

Heat

The following questions are about exercise in the heat:

Have you ever become ill while exercising in the heat?	No ❑	Yes ❑
Have you ever been diagnosed with heat exhaustion, heat stroke or hyperthermia?	No ❑	Yes ❑
Do you get frequent muscle cramps while exercising?	No ❑	Yes ❑
Have you ever had electrolyte (salt) or fluid imbalance?	No ❑	Yes ❑

Medical

Do you have any ongoing medical conditions or illness?	No ❑	Yes ❑

Do you have, or have you ever had any symptoms of medical problems such as:

Infections mononucleosis (**mono**), flu like symptoms or viral illness within the past month?	No ❑	Yes ❑
Disease of the **ears** (infections, hearing loss, pain), **nose** (sneezing, itchy nose, sinusitis, blocked nose) or **throat** (sore throat, hoarse voice, swollen glands in the neck)?	No ❑	Yes ❑
Blood disorders such as anemia, low iron stores, sickle cell trait or sickle cell disease, abnormal bleeding or clotting disorder, blood clot (embolus), or other blood disorder?	No ❑	Yes ❑
Immune system including current infections, recurrent infections, HIV/AIDS, leukemia, or are you using any immunosuppressive medication?	No ❑	Yes ❑
Skin problems such as rashes, infections (fungus, herpes, MRSA) or other skin problems?	No ❑	Yes ❑
Kidney or bladder disease, blood in the urine, loin pain, kidney stones, frequent urination, or burning during urination?	No ❑	Yes ❑
Gastrointestinal disease including heartburn, nausea, vomiting, abdominal pain, weight loss or gain (> 5kg), a change in bowel habits, chronic diarrhea, blood in the stools, or past history of liver, pancreatic or gallbladder disease?	No ❑	Yes ❑
Nervous system including past history of stroke or transient ischaemic attack (TIA), frequent or severe headaches, dizziness, blackouts, epilepsy, depression, anxiety attacks, muscle weakness, nerve tingling, loss of sensation, muscle cramps, or chronic fatigue?	No ❑	Yes ❑
Metabolic or hormonal disease including diabetes mellitus, thyroid gland disorders, or hypoglycemia (low blood sugar)?	No ❑	Yes ❑
Infections such as meningitis, hepatitis (jaundice), or chicken pox?	No ❑	Yes ❑
Arthritis or joint pain, swelling and redness not related to injury?	No ❑	Yes ❑
Were you born without, or are you **missing** a kidney, an eye or any other organ?	No ❑	Yes ❑
An **injury** to the any internal organs such as your liver, spleen, kidney(s) or lung?	No ❑	Yes ❑
Have you ever had **surgery**? (explain)	No ❑	Yes ❑
Do you get motion sickness (car, air or sea sickness)?	No ❑	Yes ❑
Do you have any other medical problems?	No ❑	Yes ❑

Family

Do any of your family members have a history of any of the following conditions (in male relatives < 55 years, female relatives < 65 years):

	No	Yes
Sudden death for no apparent reason (including drowning, unexplained car accident, or sudden infant death syndrome)?	No ❏	Yes ❏
Unexplained fainting, seizures, or near drowning?	No ❏	Yes ❏
Died before age 50 due to heart disease?	No ❏	Yes ❏
Disability or symptoms from heart disease before age 50?	No ❏	Yes ❏
Other heart problems including electrical problems (arrhythmia) or heart enlargement, cardiomyopathy, heart surgery, pacemaker or defibulator?	No ❏	Yes ❏
High blood pressure or high blood cholesterol?	No ❏	Yes ❏
Marfan's Syndrome?	No ❏	Yes ❏
Bleeding disorder, Sickle cell trait or sickle cell disease?	No ❏	Yes ❏
Tuberculosis or Hepatitis?	No ❏	Yes ❏
Anaesthetic reaction or problem?	No ❏	Yes ❏
Other condition such as stroke, diabetes, cancer, arthritis (describe)?	No ❏	Yes ❏
Are you unsure of your family history?	No ❏	Yes ❏

Medications

The following questions are about medications and supplements you are taking, or have taken in the past month:

	No	Yes
Medications that have been prescribed by a doctor (include insulin, allergy shots or pills, sleeping pills, anti-inflammatory medications etc.)?	No ❏	Yes ❏
Non-prescription medications (include pain killers, anti-inflammatories, etc.)?	No ❏	Yes ❏
Vitamin or mineral **supplements** or herbal medicines?	No ❏	Yes ❏
Other substance to improve your athletic performance (include substances like creatine, weight gain products, amino acids, etc.)?	No ❏	Yes ❏
Have you ever been offered or encouraged to use **banned performance enhancing drugs**?	No ❏	Yes ❏

Allergies

Do you have any allergies to:

	No	Yes
Medication?	No ❏	Yes ❏
Anything else, such as foods, pollens, stinging insects, any plant material or any animal material?	No ❏	Yes ❏

Immunization

Indicate which immunizations you have received:

Tetanus / Diptheria (Td or Tdap)? No❏ Yes ❏: Last shot? _____

Measles / Mumps / Rubella (2 shots)? No❏ Yes ❏

Chicken Pox (Varicella)? No❏ Yes ❏

Meningitis (Menimune or Menactra)? No❏ Yes ❏

Hepatitis A (2 shots)? No❏ Yes ❏

Hepatitis B (3 shots)? No❏ Yes ❏

Malaria? No❏ Yes ❏

Have you had a TB Test (PPD)? No❏ Yes ❏ Result? _____

Have you had any other immunizations? No❏ Yes ❏ Explain: _____

Female

These questions are for females only:

	No	Yes
Have you ever had a menstrual period?	No ❏	Yes ❏
What was your age at your first menstrual period?: _____		
Do you have regular menstrual cycles?	No ❏	Yes ❏
How many menstrual cycles did you have in the last year?: _____		
When was your most recent menstrual period?: _____		
Have you had a stress fracture in the past?	No ❏	Yes ❏
Have you ever been identified as having a problem with your bones such as low bone density (osteopenia or osteoporosis)?	No ❏	Yes ❏
Are you presently taking any female hormones (estrogen, progesterone, birth control pills)?	No ❏	Yes ❏
Have you ever had a sexually transmitted disease such as gonorrhea, syphilis, venereal warts, chlamydia or other infection?	No ❏	Yes ❏

Male

These questions are for males only:

	No	Yes
Do you have two normal testicles?	No ❏	Yes ❏
Have you ever had a hernia or swelling around the testicle (varicocele, hydrocele)?	No ❏	Yes ❏
Have you ever had an injury to a testicle?	No ❏	Yes ❏
Have you ever had surgery for an undescended testicle, testicular injury or problem?	No ❏	Yes ❏
Have you ever had a sexually transmitted disease such as gonorrhea, syphilis, venereal warts, chlamydia or other infection?	No ❏	Yes ❏

Head & Neck

Have you ever had any of the following problems related to your head or neck?:

	No	Yes
Eye injury, or other problems with your vision?	No ❏	Yes ❏
Headaches with exercise?	No ❏	Yes ❏
Have you ever had numbness, tingling or weakness in your arms and legs or been unable to move your arms or legs after being hit or falling?	No ❏	Yes ❏
Do you have, or have you been x-rayed for, neck (atlantoaxial) instability?	No ❏	Yes ❏
Have you had an injury to your teeth?	No ❏	Yes ❏
Do you have any other decayed, missing or filled teeth?	No ❏	Yes ❏
Do you have a dental prosthesis or appliance?	No ❏	Yes ❏
Have you had your wisdom teeth removed?	No ❏	Yes ❏

Injury

Have you ever had an injury to your face, head, skull or brain (including a concussion, confusion, memory loss or headache from a hit to your head, having your "bell rung" or getting "dinged")?	No ❏	Yes ❏

Have you had a problem or an injury like a sprain, strain, muscle or ligament tear, or tendonitis, broken bone, stress fracture or joint injury (that caused you to miss a practice or competition) to any of the following areas of your body?

	No	Yes
Neck or spine (including a "stinger," or "whiplash,")	No ❏	Yes ❏
Upper back (thoracic spine)	No ❏	Yes ❏
Lower back (lumbar spine)	No ❏	Yes ❏
Chest and ribs	No ❏	Yes ❏
Shoulder area (including collar bone)	No ❏	Yes ❏
Upper arm	No ❏	Yes ❏

Elbow	No ☐	Yes ☐
Lower arm (forearm)	No ☐	Yes ☐
Wrist	No ☐	Yes ☐
Hand or fingers	No ☐	Yes ☐
Pelvis, groin or hip (including sports hernia)	No ☐	Yes ☐
Thigh (including hamstrings and quadriceps)	No ☐	Yes ☐
Knee	No ☐	Yes ☐
Lower leg (calf or shin)	No ☐	Yes ☐
Ankle	No ☐	Yes ☐
Foot, heel or toes	No ☐	Yes ☐

Other

Tests - If not already mentioned above, have you had any other tests, for any injury or condition including blood tests, X-rays, MRI, CT scan, Bone scan, Ultrasound, Electroencephalogram (EEG), Electromyogram (EMG), Nerve conduction studies (NCS), Electrocardiogram (ECG/EKG), Echocardiogram (Echo), Exercise stress test or other tests?   No ☐   Yes ☐

Treatment - If not already mentioned above, have you ever received any of the following treatments for any condition?

Surgery?	No ☐	Yes ☐
Been prescribed a **brace, sling, cast, walking boot, orthotic, crutches** or other appliance?	No ☐	Yes ☐
Cortisone injection?	No ☐	Yes ☐
Been prescribed other **rehabilitation or therapy**?	No ☐	Yes ☐
Have you ever spent the night **in a hospital** or been admitted to a hospital as an inpatient or outpatient?	No ☐	Yes ☐
Been referred to a **medical specialist** (cardiologist, neurologist or other medical person) for any condition not already mentioned?	No ☐	Yes ☐

Equipment

Do you wear eye glasses or contact lenses?	No ☐	Yes ☐
Are you **currently** using any of the following protective equipment?	No ☐	Yes ☐
Do you use protective eyewear?	No ☐	Yes ☐
Special equipment (pads, braces, etc.)?	No ☐	Yes ☐
Mouth guard for sports?	No ☐	Yes ☐
If you wear a **helmet** for sports, how old is it?	No ☐	Yes ☐

Nutrition

The following questions are about nutrition:

Do you worry about your weight or body composition?	No ☐	Yes ☐
Are you satisfied with your eating pattern?	No ☐	Yes ☐
Are you a vegetarian?	No ☐	Yes ☐
Do you lose weight to meet weight requirements for your sport?	No ☐	Yes ☐
Does your weight affect the way that you feel about yourself?	No ☐	Yes ☐
Do you worry that you have lost control over how much you eat?	No ☐	Yes ☐
Do you make yourself sick when you are uncomfortably full?	No ☐	Yes ☐
Do you ever eat in secret?	No ☐	Yes ☐
Do you currently suffer or have you ever suffered in the past with an eating disorder?	No ☐	Yes ☐
What is your current weight?	No ☐	Yes ☐
How tall are you without shoes?	No ☐	Yes ☐

Discuss

Do you have any other concerns that you would like to discuss with a doctor?	No ☐	Yes ☐

Explain "YES" answers here:

```



```

I hereby state that, to the best of my knowledge, my answers to the above questions are complete and correct.

Signature of athlete: _____

Signature of parents or legal representative (when needed): _____ Date _____

Source: Ljungqvist et al, (2009); Reprinted with permission from IOC Consensus Statement on Periodic Health Evaluation of the Elite Athlete (2009).

References

Ainsworth BE, Haskell WL, Herrmann SD, *et al.* (2011) 2011 Compendium of Physical Activities: a second update of codes and MET values. *Med Sci Sports Exerc*, 43(8), 1575–1581.

Dusek T. (2001) Influence of high intensity training on menstrual cycle disorders in athletes. *Croat Med J*, 42(1), 79–82.

Gibbs JC, Nattiv A, Barrack MT, *et al.* (2013) Low bone density risk is higher in exercising women with multiple Triad risk factors. *Med Sci Sports Exerc*, 46(1), 167–176.

IOC Consensus Statement on Periodic Health Evaluation of the Elite Athlete. 2009. (http://www.olympic.org/assets/importednews/documents/en_report_1448.pdf) (accessed on November 17, 2013).

Ljungqvist A, Jenoure PJ, Engebretsen L, *et al.* (2009) The International Olympic Committee (IOC) consensus statement on periodic health evaluation of elite athletes, March 2009. *Clin J Sport Med*, 19(5), 347–365.

Misra M, Katzman D, Miller KK, *et al.* (2011) Physiologic estrogen replacement increases bone density in adolescent girls with anorexia nervosa. *J Bone Miner Res*, 26(10), 2430–2438.

Nattiv A, Loucks AB, Manore MM, *et al.* (2007) American College of Sports Medicine position stand. The female athlete triad. *Med Sci Sports Exerc*, 39(10), 1867–1882.

Sundgot-Borgen J and Torstveit MK. (2004) Prevalence of eating disorders in elite athletes is higher than in the general population. *Clin J Sport Med*,14(1), 25–32.

Recommended reading

Barrack MT, Ackerman KE, and Gibbs JC. (2013) Update on the female athlete triad. *Curr Rev Musculoskelet Med*, 6(2), 195–204.

De Souza MJ, Nattiv A, Joy E, *et al.* (2014) 2014 Female Athlete Triad Coalition Consensus Statement on Treatment and Return to Play of the Female Athlete Triad: 1st International Conference held in San Francisco, California, May 2012 and 2nd International Conference held in Indianapolis, Indiana, May 2013. *Clin J Sport Med*, 24(2), 96–119.

IOC Medical Commission Position Stand on the Female Athlete Triad, http://www.olympic.org/assets/importednews/documents/en_report_917.pdf (accessed on November 17, 2013).

Mountjoy M, Sundgot-Borgen J, Burke L, *et al.* (2014) IOC Consensus Statement. Beyond the Triad – RED-S in sport. *Br J Sports Med*. 48, 491–497.

Chapter 10
Hyperandrogenism and gender change

Martin Ritzén

Department of Women's and Children's Health, Karolinska Institutet, Stockholm, Sweden

Introduction

In almost all sports, the athletes are divided into two categories: male and female. Early on, this categorization may have had its roots in the belief that women were too fragile to expose themselves to heavy exercise. Women were therefore forbidden to take part in very strenuous activities. For example, the very popular 90-km Swedish ski race "Vasaloppet" was until 1981 out of bounds for women, in spite of protests from able women skiers. A TV interview of a competitor at that time revealed that the moustache-carrying competitor was a woman, masquerading as a male! She did so well in the race that the organizers later were forced to accept women as unofficial participants. Not until 1997 were the women fully accepted. They now ski together with the men, but the results are listed separately.

Today, almost all sports arrange competitions for both men and women—but always in separate categories. Horseback events seem to be the exception. Why are the two sexes separated in all other sports?

The simple answer is that the average man is stronger and faster than the average woman. This is true also at the highest elite level, where both men and women are professionals and undergo strenuous full-time training to get to the top. This is obvious for the true strength-dependent events (weight lifting, boxing, etc.) but also in running; the world records are about 10% better in the male than the female category, and none of the female medallists in 2013 Athletic World Championships would have ended up among the top athletes in the male events (Table 10.1). Therefore, women in general do not want to compete against men, which necessitates rules and regulations on who is qualified to compete as a woman.

Why are males stronger and faster than women?

Men are on average about 13 cm taller than women, which gives them an advantage in many sports. But there is a major overlap between the sexes; the mean height of Swedish men is 181 cm, but the 95% confidence limits are wide (169–193 cm). Similarly, the variation around the mean height of young women (167 cm in Sweden) is between 155 and 179 cm.

It has long been accepted that anabolic/androgenic hormones can enhance physical performance. Therefore, heavy penalties are cast on those athletes, male and female, that cheat by doping themselves with such hormones. The natural difference in testosterone levels in blood of men and women is the most decisive factor that during and after puberty makes the average man to build

The Female Athlete, First Edition. Edited by Margo L. Mountjoy.
© 2015 International Olympic Committee. Published 2015 by John Wiley & Sons, Inc.

Table 10.1 Results from World Championships in Athletics, Moscow 2013. The winning woman would not have been better than number 32 in any of these events if she had competed in the men's qualification heats (100–1500 m) or finals (10000 m and marathon)

Event	Winning man	Winning woman	Best woman among men's qualification	Percent difference best man/woman
100 m	9.77 sec	10.71 sec	56	9
400 m	43.74 sec	49.41 sec	32	11
1500 m	3.36 min	4.02 min	35	11
10000 m	27.21 min	30.43 min	Last of 35	11
Marathon	2 hr 9 min	2 hr 25 min	40	11

much more muscles than the average woman. And in the case of testosterone, there is no overlap between healthy men and women (Figure 10.1). This nonoverlap is unique—no other hormone or other known factors are so discriminating between the two sexes. However, during and immediately after heavy exercise, testosterone levels increase somewhat in women and decreases in men.

Hyperandrogenism in women

Both men and women have both male and female sex hormones, although the normal levels are widely different. Estrogens are necessary for skeletal health in both sexes—a complete deficiency of estrogenic

Male and female testosterone levels

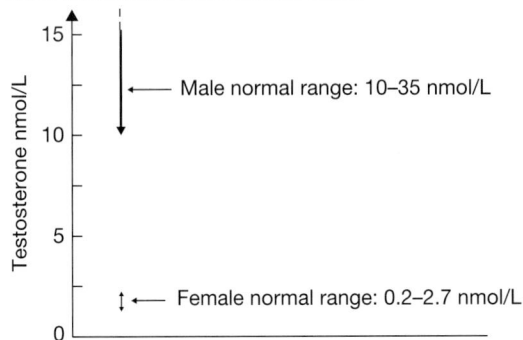

Figure 10.1 Illustration of levels of testosterone in the blood of healthy men and women. The exact values may vary a little, depending on the laboratory and the methods used. Under resting conditions, there is no overlap between the sexes.

hormones or insensitivity to them results in severe osteoporosis also in men. Furthermore, such rare men never cease growing! Similarly, small amounts of androgens from adrenals and ovaries are present in the blood of healthy women (Figure 10.1), although an androgen deficiency in women does not manifest itself by severe symptoms.

For women, a major increase in testosterone levels in blood will lead to more or less pronounced virilization, with increased hair growth over the pubic, axillary and facial areas, acne, male sweat odour, deepening of the voice, increased clitoral size, and increased muscle volume and strength. This condition with increased levels of testosterone in blood is called *hyperandrogenism*, which can be caused not only by a number of inborn errors in the metabolism of steroid hormones, but also by acquired diseases later in life. However, the tissues must also be able to respond to the androgens to elicit a response. In rare instances, this response is diminished or absent; the individual has the so-called "Complete or Partial Androgen Insensitivity Syndrome (CAIS or PAIS)," and consequently little or no benefit from the elevated testosterone levels.

Causes of hyperandrogenism in women

All *de novo* steroid hormone synthesis occurs in either the adrenals or the gonads (ovaries and testes). Thus, diseases that affect these organs sometimes results in increased production of testosterone, in both women and men. Such diseases may be acquired in postnatal life (steroid-producing tumours, abnormal regulation of steroid synthesis as in polycystic ovary syndrome, PCOS), or they may be due to inborn errors of steroid hormone synthesis or metabolism. Examples of such disorders are listed in Table 10.2. If the sensitivity to androgens is normal, the increased testosterone levels will lead to virilization of women and as a result of that, increased muscle mass and an advantage in sport when competing against other women.

PCOS is a very common ovarian disorder that among other symptoms includes increased levels of testosterone, sometimes as high as 5 nmol/L (to be compared to up to 2.7 nmol/L in healthy women). Because of its high incidence, it can almost to be regarded as a normal variant, and the increased testosterone levels must be accepted also in sport.

Congenital adrenal hyperplasia (CAH) is caused by inborn errors of steroid metabolism that are due to deficiencies in certain enzymes in the adrenal cortex. If the deficiency is severe, it is life-threatening. Milder forms survive, but at the expense of sometimes markedly elevated androgen levels in blood. Girls born with severe CAH are more or less virilized, sometimes to the extent that they are thought to be boys and raised as such. After diagnosis and proper treatment with hydrocortisone (or another glucocorticoid) and salt-retaining hormone, they live a normal life. However, if the

glucocorticoid is under-dosed, androgen production will again rise.

Foetuses with **5α-reductase type 2 deficiency** cannot convert testosterone to dihydrotestosterone (DHT) during foetal life, which is necessary for masculine development of external genitalia (penis and scrotum). XY foetuses will therefore, in spite of testicles and normal testosterone production for a boy, most often be brought up as girls. In puberty and adulthood, however, an isoenzyme (5α-reductase type 1) will be activated, and virilization will proceed. The testosterone levels in blood reach male levels, which gives these women a definite advantage in competition with other women.

XY individuals with **androgen insensitivity syndrome** will also be born with insufficient development of male external genitalia. In its complete form (CAIS), the androgen insensitivity prevents male development altogether and the child is born with normal female external genitalia. If some sensitivity remains (PAIS), partial masculinization will occur. The degree of male development at birth is instrumental for the choice of gender— male or female. Those with so poor masculinization at birth that they are assigned female sex will not show any major virilization at puberty either. Thus, both women with CAIS and PAIS have no or little benefit in sport from their (for a woman) high

Table 10.2 Some benign conditions that lead to hyperandrogenism in women

Condition	Incidence	Comments	Advantage in sports?
Polycystic ovary syndrome (PCOS)	5–10%	In adults, testosterone levels often exceed the range for healthy women	Yes
Congenital adrenal hyperplasia (CAH)	Classic form 1/12 000 Nonclassic form 1/150?	XX. Classic form: virilized at birth. Nonclassic form: not virilized at birth. May be undiagnosed	Yes, but only if undertreated
5α-reductase type 2 deficiency	Very rare	XY individuals may be assigned female sex. At puberty, virilization proceeds	Yes
Complete androgen insensitivity (CAIS)	1/50 000?	XY. Completely female external genitalia. As adults, they have high testosterone, without effect	No
Partial androgen insensitivity (PAIS)	1/30 000?	XY. Ambiguous at birth. If the testes are in place, testosterone production may give moderate androgen signs at puberty	No
Ovotesticular DSD	Very rare	XX or XY. Have both ovaries and testes. Born with ambiguous genitalia. Virilization continues in puberty	Yes
Aromatase deficiency	Extremely rare	XX individuals are born virilized. Virilization continues at and after puberty.	Yes

testosterone levels in blood. Patients with PAIS are at increased risk of developing testicular tumours.

Women with **ovotesticular disorder of sex development** develop both testicular and ovarian tissues. Testosterone production during foetal life is subnormal for a male, excessive for a female. Therefore, external genitalia are found to be ambiguous at birth leading to uncertainty in the decision of sex or rearing. At puberty, testosterone (and estrogen) production resumes, and women may be virilized.

In **aromatase deficiency**, the foetus, including the placenta, is unable to convert foetal androgens to estrogens. This leads to the accumulation of androgens and virilization of girls, both in utero and in puberty and adulthood.

Understanding the inborn causes of hyperandrogenism requires some knowledge of the normal and abnormal development of the sex organs during foetal life. This will be summarized below.

Normal and abnormal sex development

During early embryonic life, the primitive gonad differentiates into either an ovary or a testicle. This is the key moment for future development; absence of testicular development will lead to female genital organs, while a testis will produce hormones that direct male development. A foetus without gonads will develop like a normal female. The primitive gonad will develop into a testis, provided that certain genes are present and active, the most important being the SRY gene, located on the Y chromosome. The foetal ovary is not important for normal development of female genitalia, including vagina, uterus, and oviducts. A schematic picture of foetal sex differentiation is shown in Figure 10.2.

The sex chromosome constitution XY and XX are linked to male and female differentiation, respectively. However, the important genes of these chromosomes that direct male gonadal differentiation (SRY on the Y chromosome and the androgen receptor gene, AR, on the X chromosome) can be mutated and more or less nonfunctional. An XY foetus with a nonfunctional androgen receptor will not respond to testosterone or DHT and therefore develops like a female—except for the uterus and oviducts that will be suppressed by the normal testicular production of AMH. An inborn nonfunctioning 5α-reductase type II gene is of particular interest for the issue of hyperandrogenism in adulthood: During foetal life, this deficiency will prevent the normal male differentiation of

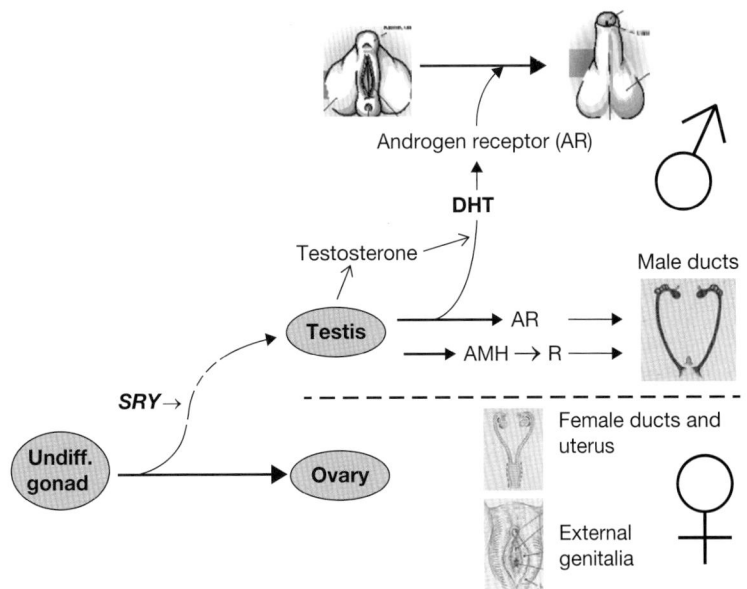

Figure 10.2 A simplified schematic representation of normal sex differentiation. The early development of the primitive gonad into a testis will direct further male development: Testosterone secretion by the testis will act directly to develop the male internal genital ducts and, after conversion to DHT by the enzyme 5α-reductase type II, the external genitalia (penis and scrotum). A normal receptor for androgenic (AR) is essential for the action of both testosterone and DHT. Testicular secretion of anti-Müllarian hormone (AMH) suppresses the female duct system. In the absence of testes, female genitalia will develop.

external genitalia by DHT (see Figure 10.2) and the child appears female at birth. However, from puberty and on, the testes will resume testosterone production and (through the action of an isoenzyme, 5α-reductase type I) form DHT, which has full action on the body (including muscles) and cause sometimes severe virilization. In the presence of male levels of testosterone, muscles may develop like those of a man rather than a woman.

Definitions of male or female sex

Most people think that it is easy to define the sex of a person; the anatomy of the genital organs at birth decides the sex. This is the rule, but there are many exceptions.

Sex can be defined from different aspects: the assigned sex, the chromosomal sex, the hormonal sex, and the sex identity. A chain of events during embryonic development must work in synchrony to end up in clear-cut male or female anatomy at birth. If any link in this chain is broken, it may be difficult to assign male or female sex at birth—the sex is uncertain due to a disorder of sex development (DSD) ending up as an *intersex* condition. But in most cultures, society demands a decision—male or female. Later in life, the decision may turn out to be wrong. Also, in some individuals with a normal male or female anatomy, a person may instinctively feel that his or her sex does not agree with the development of the body, and decide to change sex in adulthood (*transsexuals*). Both DSDs and transsexuals may cause confusion when it comes to defining males and females in sport. They will be dealt with separately in this chapter.

Short history of gender issues in sport

At a time when little was known about abnormal sex differentiation, masculine-looking female athletes were sometimes suspected to be masquerading males. A well-known example is Stella Walsh, "the fastest woman in the world." She won medals in both the 1932 and 1936 Olympic Games but had to live with rumours that she was actually a man. Many years later, long after her athletic career was ended, she was killed in a road accident and an autopsy revealed that she had an XY intersex condition. Similarly, the German 1936 champion in high jump Dora Ratjen later changed sex to male. These cases and others prompted the British Women's Amateur Athletic Association to request in 1948 some sort of "Sex certificate," and later, at some competitions, physical examination ("nude parade") was requested to prove the female sex. This, of course, caused protests, and in 1968, it was instead thought that testing for X chromatin in buccal cells would reveal the "true" sex. However, this method also failed, as demonstrated by the case of the Spanish athlete Maria Patino, who later wrote a book about her experiences. In 1985, she passed one such test but failed a second one and was disqualified. She is completely insensitive to androgens and therefore had no advantage of androgenic hormones—and still she was humiliated in public and her medals were withdrawn for three years. The IAAF then accepted that chromosomal sex does not always go along with the assigned sex and abandoned all testing. But the IOC in 1992 instead changed to testing for the SRY gene, specific for the Y chromosome, until finally, in 1999, also the IOC gave up genetic testing. By then, it had been known for a long time that some women can carry a Y chromosome without any signs of masculinity and therefore have no advantage in sports. After that, there were no regulations on how to handle gender issues in international competitions.

The media were still fascinated by rumours that some women athletes were "really" males. The worst example in recent time was the way media handled the case when Caster Semenya clearly won the 800 meter World Championship in Berlin in 2009. The IAAF was taken by surprise and had no policy to follow and announced that "a sex investigation" would be performed. No medical expertise was available to educate the IAAF that sex identity cannot be determined by hormonal or genetic tests, but is intrinsic to the person herself. After that scandal, both IAAF and IOC sat down to work out regulations and rules to follow for female athletes that want to compete with other women.

The present regulations of hyperandrogenism in women's sport

In 2011, the IAAF published new guidelines, the most important feature of which is that the sex of a person must never be questioned. However, it was acknowledged that some women born and raised as girls have so high testosterone production that it gives them a muscular physiology like a man. Focus was now shifted to the levels of testosterone in blood, not on the sex or gender. As described above, under resting conditions, the testosterone concentration in blood shows no overlap between men and women. It was therefore declared that women who have testosterone levels in the male range (for simplicity defined as >10 nmol/L) and normal sensitivity to androgenic hormones would not be eligible to compete in the female category. If treatment of the underlying condition brings down the testosterone levels below the male range, the woman can return to competition. The new regulations including explanatory notes can be found on the IAAF homepage.

The IOC issued similar rules and regulations for women with hyperandrogenism in 2012, to be executed before and during the London Olympic Games. Some but not all international sports federations have also instituted similar rules for their respective areas.

Both the IAAF and the IOC stress that the regulations are "living documents" that will be updated as the scientific understanding of hyperandrogenism in sports advances.

Male-to-female sex change

Occasionally, men that change sex from male to female want to compete within their new gender. Therefore, the IOC called for an expert meeting in 2003 that resulted in the so-called "Stockholm consensus on sex reassignment in sports." First, it was concluded that for those that change sex before puberty, no special ruling was needed—they should automatically be eligible to compete in their new sex. However, if the change is

done during or after puberty, the issue is more complicated, since in male-to-female transition at a time when the male sex hormones have already made their imprint on the muscle mass, a certain period of time should pass between the removal of the testicles and the return to competition, now in the female category. Based on the studies on the rate of regression of muscle volume in male-to-female transsexuals, it was concluded that two years should pass between change of legal sex and being allowed to compete as females. At the time of the Stockholm consensus, most countries required gonadectomy before changing the legal sex, so this was written into the rules. Other requirements for eligibility for male-to-female transsexuals to compete as females were legal recognition as well as hormonal therapy appropriate for their assigned sex.

However, the attitude to sex change is changing rapidly. Today, the requirement of castration and other genital surgery for change of legal sex has been abandoned in some countries. The IOC now acknowledges that the "Stockholm consensus" is due for revision. More recently, the IAAF in 2011 issued regulations for male-to-female sex reassignment and sports. The only formal requirements are documentation of legal change of sex and testosterone levels in blood and urine that must not be in the male range. Gonadectomy is not mentioned. Thus, the regulation for transsexuals is coming close to that for hyperandrogenism.

Conclusions

In most sports, men and women compete in different categories, since men on average have a body build that make them outperform women in sports. Therefore, a clear definition of who is eligible to compete in the women's category is needed. Although it may seem easy to tell a man from a woman, rare exceptions cause intermediate sex development and make clear definitions necessary. In the past, genetic tests were thought to be objective means for separating men from women. However, some men can have female (XX) and some women male (XY) sex chromosomes.

One major and easily identifiable cause of the stronger body of men is the male production and action of testosterone during puberty and in adulthood. Testosterone is a major factor in building muscles. During resting and healthy conditions, there is no overlap between male and female levels of testosterone in blood. This knowledge has now been adopted by the IOC and the IAAF; in the present ruling of eligibility to compete in the women's category, testosterone levels in blood rather than chromosomal or gonadal sex is the dividing line: If a woman with normal sensitivity to androgens has testosterone levels in blood that are in the normal male range, she is not eligible to compete with other women until the levels have been reduced. The cause of such (for a woman) abnormally high testosterone concentrations in blood may be acquired or inborn, the latter due to genetic abnormalities.

Men with the so-called "gender dysphoria" (transsexualism) may decide to change to female gender. If this change occurs in adulthood, the persisting male musculature will give them an advantage in sports if they compete with other women. The present ruling by the IOC which dates from 2004 states that 2 years must pass from the time of legal change of sex (including surgery) to eligibility to compete as a woman. Recently, the requirement for castration and surgery to the new sex has been abandoned in several countries. Therefore, the IOC regulations are under revision. The IAAF in 2011 introduced similar rules, but there is no requirement for surgery in those regulations.

Recommended reading

IAAF Regulations Governing Eligibility of Females with Hyperandrogenism to Compete in Women's Competition – In force as from 1st May 2011. Updated December 11, 2012. http://www.iaaf.org/about-iaaf/documents/medical (accessed on July 15, 2014).

IOC Regulations on Female Hyperandrogenism, updated for the Solchi Games 2014. http://www.olympic.org/Documents/Commissions_PDFfiles/Medical_commission/IOC-Regulations-on-Female-Hyperandrogenism.pdf (accessed on July 15, 2014).

IOC statement on sports and sex reassignment: http://www.olympic.org/content/news/media-resources/manual-news/1999-2009/2004/05/18/ioc-approves-consensus-with-regard-to-athletes-who-have-changed-sex/

Lee PA, Houk CP, Ahmed SF, and Hughes IA. (2006) Consensus statement on management of intersex disorders. *Pediatrics*, 118, e488–e500.

Tucker R and Collins M. (2010) The science of sex verification and athletic performance. *Int J Sports Physiol Perform*, 5, 127–139.

Chapter 11

Sexual harassment and abuse in sport: implications for health care providers

Trisha Leahy[1] and Kari Fasting[2]

[1]The Hong Kong Sports Institute, Sha Tin, Hong Kong
[2]Department of Social and Cultural Studies, Norwegian School of Sport Sciences, Oslo, Norway

Introduction

Sport is an important social institution, and research documenting the public health benefits of active sporting lifestyles underpins many governmental policy initiatives promoting its development from community to elite levels. However, during the last 20 years international research documenting, the occurrence of sexual harassment and abuse in sport, has led to a more critical analysis of the quality of sporting environments and their impact on young people. Sexual harassment and abuse are social problems existing in all our societies. The sports sector, like other sectors of the community, cannot totally secure itself. What can be achieved through increasing vigilance and detererence is a minimization of risk.

The International Olympic Committee (IOC) has taken the lead on this issue and issued a consensus statement on sexual harassment and abuse in sport in 2007 specifically recognizing all the rights of athletes, including the right to enjoy a safe and supportive sport environment. This was followed by online interactive educational tools for federations, associations, athletes, and coaches in 2012. Following the IOC's publication of its position paper, the related issue of violence against children in sport

was subsequently taken up by the United Nations Children's Fund ("UNICEF") who published a review in 2010 which found that most countries do not have effectively functioning structures and system to prevent and eliminate all forms of child abuse in sport. It was further recognized that abuse prevention, child protection, and measures to safeguard the well-being of children are generally not well embedded in sport delivery systems.

Our goal in this chapter is to provide an overview for health care providers working with female athletes. We begin by defining sexual harassment and abuse and summarizing what is currently known about the prevalence in sport. We then outline the key elements of the psychological impact of sexual harassment and abuse on athletes and provide a summary of symptoms that may be observed and which may indicate possible sexual harassment or abuse experiences. Using a biopsychosocial perspective, we advocate for the active participation of all members of the athlete's entourage, including health care providers to collaborate in a multidisciplinary engagement to act as gatekeepers for athlete's safety in identifying, intervening, and acting to minimize the risk of sexual harassment and abuse of athletes in our sport systems.

Understanding sexual harassment and abuse in sport

In this chapter, we focus on sexual forms of harassment and abuse even though we recognize that different forms of harassment and abuse also occur. Sexual harassment refers to behavior toward an individual or group that involves sexualized verbal, nonverbal, or physical behavior, whether intended or unintended, legal or illegal, which is experienced by the victim as unwanted. Verbal sexual harassment may be unwanted intimate questions relating to body, clothes, or one's private life, "jokes" with a sexual innuendo, and proposals or demands for sexual services or sexual relationships. These may also be in the form of unwanted telephone calls, text messages or letters with a sexual content. Nonverbal sexual harassment may be for instance: staring, showing pictures of objects with sexual allusions. Physical sexual harassment on the other hand can be unwanted or unnecessary physical contact of a sexual nature, such as "pinching," pressing against another's body, or attempting to kiss or caress another person.

Behaviors that are characterized as sexual harassment may also be considered as sexual abuse depending on the context, such as severity, the age of the victim, and the local legal system. Sexual abuse involves any sexual activity where consent is not or cannot be given. This includes sexual contact accomplished by force or the threat of force, regardless of the age of the victim or perpetrator. Any sexual activity between an adult and a child regardless of whether there is deception, or the child understands the sexual nature of the activity, is considered to be sexual abuse. Child sexual abuse can also include noncontact (e.g., exhibitionism, involving a child in sexually explicit conversation, engaging a child in pornographic photography), contact (sexual touching, masturbation), and penetrative (oral, vaginal, anal penetration) acts.

The occurrence of sexual harassment and abuse in sport has been documented by researchers in a number of countries during the past 15 years. Research in the area began with both prevalence studies and qualitative investigations of athletes' experiences, but there is a marked variety of approaches to the subject, both theoretical and methodological. Prevalence rates suggested by research reports across different countries vary according to definitions and research design, making it difficult to compare data across studies. Nevertheless, indicative figures suggest prevalence rates of between 19% and 92 % for sexual harassment in sport and between 2% and 49% for sexual abuse.

Research also indicates that sexual harassment and abuse seem to occur across all sports regardless of athlete gender. Whereas sexual harassment appears, in general, to be perpetrated more frequently by peers, studies also indicate that perpetrators of sexual abuse within sports systems are primarily persons in positions of authority, trust, or guardianship, including coaches and less frequently, officials, support staff, and peers. Recent studies from Africa appear to indicate that even for sexual abuse, the frequency of peer abuse may be much higher than previously reported in other studies.

Most studies to date have taken place in Europe, the United States, Canada, and Australia, and it is only very recently that articles have been published from Africa and Asia. Recent figures from Japan indicate comparable (30%) prevalence rates of reported sexual harassment by female athletes. Also consistent with previous research findings, international level female athletes in the Japan study reported higher rates of sexual harassment in sport.

We have until recently only had anecdotal information about the prevalence and experiences of sexual harassment and abuse among athletes in Africa. One master's thesis which studied the situation in Tanzania found a prevailing perception among sport leaders that sexual harassment and abuse did occur in sport to such an extent that parents found it problematic to send their daughters to sport training. A more extensive survey in Zimbabwe reported high percentages of reported sexual harassment and abuse, with 84% of the athletes reporting that they had experienced severe sexual harassment and 49% reporting that they had experienced sexual abuse, raising additional concerns about the risk of HIV and AIDS in those communities.

The psychological impact of sexual harassment and abuse

The psychological impact of sexual harassment and abuse varies considerably among individuals depending on the characteristics of the harassment or abuse experience itself (e.g., duration, frequency, invasiveness, violence, relationship of the perpetrator to the victim); characteristics of the victim (e.g., age at onset, other traumatic experiences, history of maltreatment), and the characteristics of social support provided to the victim, with positive social support correlating with significantly better adjustment. In general, and particularly where the harassment and abuse is prolonged and repeated and perpetrated by those in positions of trust, guardianship, or authority, as is often the case in sport contexts, a trauma framework provides an appropriate context for treatment interventions. A detailed discussion of the complex psychological sequelae of sexual harassment and abuse is beyond the scope of this article, and any treatment intervention requires specific psychological or psychiatric expertise. Nevertheless, a summary of commonly observed symptoms is provided below to enable health care providers working with female athletes to be alert to possible indicators of sexual harassment and abuse.

From a trauma perspective, posttraumatic stress disorder and dissociation are often observed as primary responses to trauma. Core posttraumatic symptoms include reexperiencing (e.g., intrusive thoughts, nightmares), avoidance (e.g., of thoughts, feelings, places, or people associated with the trauma) and hyperarousal (e.g., physiological reactivity to trauma cues, hypervigilance). Dissociation involves a splitting between the "observing self" and the "experiencing self." During a traumatic experience, dissociation provides protective detachment from overwhelming affect and pain, but if it persists, it can result in severe disruption within the usually integrated functions of consciousness, memory, identity, or perception of the environment. This is expressed by an athlete recalling her junior career during which she was sexually abused by her coach: "I can't really remember much of it. It's as if it happened to someone else, or, as if I wasn't there."

A number of interrelated, or secondary trauma-based symptoms in physical, emotional, cognitive, and relational domains, have been observed in survivors of prolonged and repeated sexual harassment and abuse. In the physical domain, somatization and functional medical conditions are often reported, with resulting injury and inability to maintain training loads. Other negative health consequences that have been reported include headaches, sleep disturbance, weight loss or gain,

gastrointestinal disturbances and nausea, fatigue, neck and back pain. For example, an athlete who was sexually harassed reported, referring to such physical symptoms:

> When I read my diary that I wrote ten years ago, I realize that the same things are bothering me today. This disturbs me, makes me nervous, anxious and makes it difficult to sleep.

In the emotional domain, an inability to regulate the intensity of affective responses (affect dysregulation), as well as depression, anxiety, grief, and fear has been reported. For example, one athlete said:

> I literally had breakdowns when I was training, and that was the way I'd release the tension and emotion, and other times I would try to throw my emotions against my training ability to overcome how bad I was feeling, and tell myself I've got to train harder, do more...

In the cognitive domain, alterations in attention and consciousness leading to dissociative symptoms have been observed. Self-concept can also be affected and a self-perception embedded in a sense of guilt, shame, and responsibility for the abuse is often reported. This is reflected in the words of a female athlete sexually abused by her coach for many years, "I had always accepted that it was my fault. I was too trusting, and I didn't really see it coming. I deserved to be punished." Attributions centering on hopelessness and despair may also be observed, as poignantly expressed by a female athlete abused for many years by her coach, "I felt like I was just this disease... I'd look in the mirror and have a complete feeling of emptiness." A Paralympian female athlete who had experienced long-term sexual harassment from the coach and male members of the team said, "I felt like an animal, not a human being."

In the relational domain, a very challenging and often misunderstood symptom is traumatized attachment to the perpetrator (discussed in more detail below). This refers to the situation where, the perceived powerful perpetrator's, worldview and belief system is internalized by the athlete. Traumatized attachment is particularly evident where the perpetrator is the athlete's coach ("I remember pretty much if he said jump, I'd jump. I never questioned what he said. None of us did"). Relational difficulties with trust and intimacy are also commonly observed as reported by an athlete sexually abused by her coach:

> "It's been years where I haven't been able to be close to a boy. I just don't trust them. So, for someone that I cared about, you know, I'd throw it away, because, you know, I just don't trust them."

Another athlete who was sexually harassed reported a similar difficulty:

"I don't know, you are maybe more reticent towards developing relationships with other males. One gets a bit more negative view of men in a way …I didn't have much respect for him when I left."

Trust difficulties can also extend to health care providers and other members of the support team. Trustworthiness of the health care provider may be challenged, and if not properly understood and managed, may impede the formation of a healthy, reparative relationships and treatment alliances.

The role of health care professionals in safeguarding

The athletes' accounts above illustrate the potentially serious and long-lasting effects of sexual harassment and abuse in sport. Even though specific training in psychology or psychiatry is necessary to be able to appropriately engage in therapeutic work with athletes, every health care provider working with athletes can be a part of the solution in a multidisciplinary biopsychosocial model of service provision.

A biopsychosocial framework is commonly applied within the elite sport sector, in developing gifted athletes to world-level performance standards. Within this framework, there is an assumption that biological, psychological, and social factors are integrally linked in the overall development of any athlete. Internationally, servicing infrastructures, which facilitate elite sport development, generally operate within a biopsychosocial, integrated support system targeting all aspects of each athlete's medical and physiological, psychological, social support and welfare needs. A multidisciplinary approach is a core feature of the biopsychosocial paradigm, with cross-disciplinary teams providing integrated science, and evidence-based programs and interventions to support coaching planning and programming and monitoring.

Within the biopsychosocial model therefore, health care providers are key frontline members of the athletes' entourage and, as part of the biopsychosocial, multidisciplinary support system, are in a key position to monitor the maintenance of a psychologically, physically, and sexually safe sports system in which athletes can achieve their potential. Health care providers, because of their close involvement with the team, are often the first point of contact for athletes in distress and can be an important source of support to victimized athletes. It is, therefore, important that health care providers working with athletes are aware of sport environment risk factors, in order to be able to effectively act as gatekeepers of athletes' safety in terms of prevention, and to ensure early intervention.

Understanding sport environment risk factors

While the risk factors for abuse of any kind are well documented in the medical literature, in relation to athletes' experiences of sexual harassment and abuse in sport, there are two sport environment systemic risk factors that require understanding if we are to act effectively as gatekeepers of athlete safety. These include the normalization of what might constitute psychologically abusive coaching practices, and a socio-cultural context with norms based very much on power and hierarchical relations. For example, in a recent European study among female sport students, there was a higher reported prevalence of sexual harassment experiences from athletes whose coaches demonstrated coaching behavior characterized by negative feedback, screaming, rough language, directive communication, and coach-led decision-making. The risk with this power-based method of coaching is that of overlooking and/or intruding on the athletes needs and wishes, since the athlete is left out of important processes in the relationship. An earlier Australian study had similarly reported that the normalization of psychologically abusive coaching practices had facilitated rather than challenged perpetrator strategies of grooming, controlling, and disempowering athlete victims. Where there are insufficient checks and balances on the power vested in the coach, there is a risk of creating an environment that facilitates, rather than challenges the abuse of power which is at the core of sexual harassment and abuse in sport. This is discussed below in more detail in relation to specific perpetrator methodology in sport and the bystander effect.

Perpetrator methodology in the sport environment

Sexual harassment and abuse are generally understood as abuses of power. Examples of power relations in sports include the power that people in the support network have in relation to the athletes. This especially applies to the coach, who can help young athletes achieve their sporting goals and realize their giftedness. This type of trust and power relationship is often referred to as an "expert," or "power of position" relationship. It is through the misuse of this power relationship that we see commonalities in perpetrator methodologies for sexual harassment and abuse in different studies from different countries.

The core perpetrator strategies appear to be designed to simultaneously engender feelings of powerlessness in the athlete, and conversely, to present the perpetrator as omnipotent. In cases of prolonged and repeated sexual abuse, the perpetrator imposes his/her version of reality on the athlete and successfully isolates the athlete within that reality. The perpetrator successfully maintains that reality by controlling the psychological environment, silencing, and isolating the athlete from potential sources of support. In addition to controlling the athlete's outer life, her/his inner life is controlled through direct emotional manipulation, psychological abuse, and the creation of a highly volatile, psychologically abusive training environment.

From the psychological literature, we know that the repeated imposition of a powerful perpetrator's worldview, and the lack of alternative reference points, due to isolating and silencing strategies, can result in the victim being entrapped within the perpetrator's viewpoint. In an unpredictable and volatile training environment, within the closed context of a competitive sports team, the random repetition of punishment and reward cycles can result in a feeling of extreme dependence on the perceived omnipotent perpetrator. This is what is meant by traumatized attachment to the perpetrator mentioned above. Under these conditions, disclosure will not occur, and common expectations of distress indicators will not be apparent.

The perpetrator's ability to successfully create and maintain such an environment indicates a systemic vulnerability in the sociocultural context of competitive sport (at least in some first-world countries where the research has been consistent). This context is one that has been criticized as being imbued with an intensely volatile ethos, and within which psychologically abusive coaching behaviors may be normalized as part of the winning strategy. It is this that constitutes a significant risk factor for the sports environment. This point brings us to the issue of the bystander effect.

The bystander effect

The bystander effect refers to the situation where the victim perceives that others know about, (or suspect) what is going on, but do not do anything about it. This is poignantly illustrated by a female athlete sexually abused by her coach for many years:

> He was in such a powerful position that no one interfered; I think no one questioned what he was doing. But now when I speak to people, they do say he stepped over the line with us, but...they didn't say anything. They didn't want to interfere with him (Leahy, 2010, p. 316).

Athletes' experiences of the bystander effect point to the apparent lack of systemically sanctioned accountability which allowed the perpetrator to continue for many years unchallenged by other adults in the system. Bystanders have been identified in the research as coaching, medical, psychology, and other support staff or volunteers who were not as senior in the competitive sport hierarchy as the perpetrator. The bystander effect is a risk factor that appears to be particularly acute in the elite sport context, "No one ever interfered with us because we were so elite, and no one ever questioned what we were doing" (Leahy, 2010, p. 327). Young athletes in this situation may assume that the behavior is socially acceptable, or in the case of older athletes, that the perpetrator's message that he is omnipotent is really true and that they really are trapped. This prevents disclosure.

Risk minimization

Sexual harassment and abuse are social problems, and the sports sector, similar to other sectors of the community, cannot totally secure itself. What we can perhaps achieve is to increase deterrence and decrease risk by empowering all adults in the athletes' support team, starting with ourselves as sports professionals, with the specific knowledge and resources required to understand and to act in order to empower and protect athletes and advocate for appropriate policies within the sports system.

There are four key elements to risk minimization. The first is having a well-developed code of ethics for all members of the athletes' support system. The code of ethics should explicitly articulate the behavioral guidelines for relationship and boundary management between the athletes and members of the support team. Each sport organization should also have standardized recruitment processes not only to screen job applicants suitability for the post, but also to perform criminal background checks. There should be specific job interview questions to assess applicants' knowledge and awareness of child protection, athletes' rights, and relational boundaries.

The third element, which is important to overcome the bystander effect, is comprehensive and ongoing awareness raising and education for athletes, parents, and all associated support personnel. Particularly, it is the responsibility of adults in the sports system to ensure children's safety. Education and awareness raising for athletes is also a tool to empower athletes and facilitate early disclosure. Sport organizations should have effective and supportive links with relevant local agencies that may be able to provide education and intervention assistance.

And finally, clear athlete protection policies and procedures should be in place. When sexual harassment and abuse occur in sport, it affects the athlete, the athletes' family, other members of the team, and the sport organization itself. The function of the policy is that it provides a clear organizational statement that sexual harassment and abuse will not be tolerated in the organization. It also provides a clear set of procedures for everyone to follow when a disclosure is made. This is an important step in ensuring that the organizational response does not retraumatize an already vulnerable athlete but rather acts as a positive support mechanism.

Conclusion

Those of us working in the competitive sports sector all recognize and understand the influential role of sport in the physical, psychological, and social development of young people. We acknowledge the importance of sport as a vehicle to achieve public health goals and as a bridge to link communities. However, if we are to achieve these aims, then we need to engage in a more thoughtful stewardship of sport and become part of community efforts to confront broader social issues, including sexual harassment and abuse which also occur in sport. The sport industry must become a more socially engaged sector with sports professionals using their expertise and knowledge to offer a more positive contribution to and promote athletes' welfare.

The IOC has made it clear that it is the right of all athletes to enjoy a safe and supportive sport environment and that it is in such conditions that athletes are more likely to flourish and optimize their sporting performance. Health care providers working with sports teams are in a unique position to be able to monitor the maintenance of a safe-sporting environment for athletes and to be an advocate for athletes' well-being, and the development of "a culture of dignity, respect, and safety in sport" (IOC Medical Commission, 2007).

Recommended reading

Brackenridge CH. (2001) *Spoilsports: Understanding and Preventing Sexual Exploitation in Sport*. Routledge, London.

Brackenridge CH, Fasting K, Kirby S, Leahy T, Parent S, and Svela Sand T. (2010) *The Place of Sport in the UN Study on Violence against Children*. UNICEF, Florence.

Brackenridge C, Fasting K, Kirby S, and Leahy T. (2010) *Protecting Children from Violence in Sports: A Review Focused on Industrialised Countries*. UNICEF, Florence.

Fasting K, Brackenridge C, and Knorre N. (2010) Performance level and sexual harassment prevalence among female athletes in the Czech Republic, *Women Sport Phys Act J*, 19(1), 26–32.

Fasting K, Chroni S, Hervik SE, and Knorre N. (2011) Sexual harassment in sport toward females in three European countries. *Int Rev Sociol Sport*, 46(1), 76–89.

IOC Medical Commission. (2007) Consensus statement on sexual harassment and abuse in sport. Available at http://multimedia.olympic.org/pdf/en_report_1125.pdf (accessed on December 12, 2013).

IOC Medical Commission. (2012) Sexual harassment and abuse in sport—educational tools. Available at http://www.olympic.org/sha (accessed on September, 2013).

Kirby S, Greaves L, and Hankivsky O. (2000) *The Dome of Silence: Sexual Harassment and Abuse in Sport*. Fernwood Publishing, Halifax, NS.

Leahy T. (2010) Sexual abuse in sport: implications for the sport psychology profession. In TV Ryba, RJ Schinke, and G Tenenbaum (eds), *The Cultural Turn in Sport Psychology* (pp. 315–334). Fitness Information Technology, Morgantown, WV.

Leahy T. (2008) Understanding and preventing sexual harassment and abuse in sport: implications for the sport psychology profession. *Int J Sport Exerc Psycho*, 4, 351–353.

Sand TS, Fasting K, Chroni S, Hervik SE, and Knorre N. (2011) Coaching behavior: any consequences for the prevalence of sexual harassment? *Int J Sport Sci Coach*, 6(2), 229–241.

Chapter 12
Exercise and pregnancy

Ruben Barakat[1], Alejandro Lucía[2] and Jonatan Ruiz[3]

[1]Faculty of Physical Activity and Sports Sciences, Technical University of Madrid, Spain
[2]Universidad Europea de Madrid, Spain, Instituto de Investigación Hospital 12 de Octubre (i+12), Madrid, SPAIN
[3]PROFITH "PROmoting FITness and Health through physical activity" research group, Department of Physical Education and Sport, Faculty of Sport Sciences, University of Granada, Granada, Spain

Particularities of pregnancy and childbirth

Special features of pregnancy and childbirth

Pregnancy is the unique vital process in which a woman's body control systems are modified to preserve the life of the fetus during its growth and development. Throughout 38 weeks of gestation, a women's body constantly changes to maintain body balance and biological homeostasis and deliver the baby without maternal or fetal complications. Any disarrangement or imbalance can adversely affect pregnant outcome.

But why should we exercise during pregnancy? Is there scientific evidence for a beneficial effect of regular physical activity during the course of pregnancy?

Despite pregnant woman being denied the possibility of an active gestation period in the past, there is growing evidence from observational and intervention studies that a woman with no obstetric complications may exercise during pregnancy without any detrimental impacts on maternal–fetal outcome. Fortunately, there is a current tendency toward regular physical activity during pregnancy, and more importantly, physical activity is today

considered an important part of routine daily life and the pregnancy period is no exception.

Today's concept of health has changed from the old idea of "absence of disease" to a wider concept that, besides the proper functioning of vital organs (cardio-circulatory, metabolic and hormonal functions), also considers psychological well-being and affective-social human behavior.

A sedentary lifestyle can lead to many health complications, and this also applies to pregnant women. Even Aristotle mentioned that "Difficult deliveries are due to a sedentary lifestyle" (Aristotle, C. III b.c.). Indeed, exercise is now known to benefit many aspects of a pregnant woman's health.

For a new pregnancy not to reduce quality of life, we therefore need to find (among the many options that physical activity offers) a way of avoiding a sudden decline in physical activity.

Modifications in pregnant body systems related to physical exercise

Circulatory system

Two basic facts should be taken into account:
• increased requirements due to fetal development; and
• the upward movement of certain structures as a consequence of the increased size of the uterus.

From the start of the first trimester until the end of pregnancy, cardiac output (the product of stroke volume and heart rate) increases by 30% to 40% as a

The Female Athlete, First Edition. Edited by Margo L. Mountjoy.
© 2015 International Olympic Committee. Published 2015 by John Wiley & Sons, Inc.

result of an increased heart rate (e.g., from 70 beats/min before pregnancy to 85 beats/min in late pregnancy) and a slight increase in stroke volume.

Peripheral vascular resistance diminishes, and this leads to a slight drop in blood pressure. Diastolic blood pressure decreases in the first and second trimester and returns to prepregnancy values in the third trimester. Systolic blood pressure is modified slightly, with a tendency to decrease in the first and second trimester.

Possibly the most significant (and most consequential) change during pregnancy is the compression of the inferior cava vein by the gravid uterus. When a woman adopts a supine position, this phenomenon decreases venous return to heart (Figure 12.1).

Among other factors, inferior cava vein compression affects cardiac output and variables related to the circulatory system.

Blood system

Blood volume increases by 45% (~1800 mL), and this is accounted for by both an increased plasma volume (~1500 mL) and an increased red cell volume (~350 mL). This "heme dilution" maintains adequate uteroplacental flow.

Respiratory system

Changes in the respiratory system cause anatomical and functional alterations. These modifications occur early during pregnancy owing to hormonal effects and the above-mentioned increments in blood volume, and include changes in lung dimensions and capacity as well as inspiratory/expiratory mechanisms.

Reduced functional residual capacity accompanied by increased oxygen consumption diminishes the oxygen reserve. The oxygen cost of ventilation also rises owing to an increased workload on the diaphragm. Estrogens and progesterone cause an increase in lung ventilation which gives rise to respiratory alkalosis. However, the acid–base balance is maintained by a compensatory metabolic acidosis mechanism and blood pH values remain around 7.44.

Most of these maternal breathing mechanisms are targeted at reducing arterial PCO_2 to create a mild alkalosis. This ensures maternal placental gas exchange and prevents fetal acidosis.

Metabolic processes

During pregnancy, normal metabolic processes are altered to accommodate the needs of the developing fetus. The protein contents of the body tissues increase. Carbohydrates accumulate in the liver, muscles, and placenta. In addition, fat deposits appear under the skin, especially affecting the breasts and buttocks, and this is frequently accompanied by increased blood lipid levels, including cholesterol. The pregnant woman's body accumulates the salts of several minerals that are essential for normal fetal development, that is, calcium, phosphorus, potassium and iron. In addition, hormonal changes promote water retention in the tissues.

Maternal weight gain is one of the most obvious changes that occur during pregnancy. Although there is individual variability, a weight increase from before pregnancy to the end of pregnancy of 10–13 kg is considered normal. The factors responsible for this weight gain during pregnancy are provided in Table 12.1.

Locomotor effects

Pregnant women often experience paresthesia and pain in the upper extremities as a result of marked

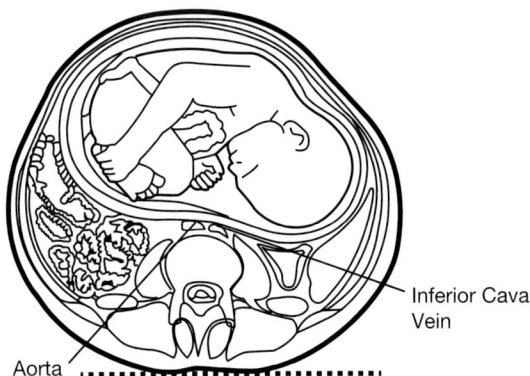

Figure 12.1 Compression of the inferior cava vein.
From De Miguel and Sanchez (2001).

Inferior Cava Vein

Aorta

Table 12.1 Maternal weight gain during pregnancy

	Maternal weight gain (grams)			
	Week 10	Week 20	Week 30	Week 40
Fetus	5	300	1500	3400
Placenta	20	170	430	650
Amniotic fluid	30	350	750	800
Uterus	140	320	600	970
Breast	45	180	360	405
Blood	100	600	1300	1250
Interstitial fluid	0	30	80	1680
Fat deposits	310	2050	3480	3345
Total gain	650	4000	8500	12 500

sinking of the cervical lordosis and shoulder girdle, frequently in the third trimester. In effect, an important characteristic of the pregnant body is the arching of the lower back or "hyperlordosis of pregnancy." This problem was traditionally attributed to the growth of the uterus, but current scientific evidence indicates that the mother offsets the deviation of her center of gravity by moving backward the entire skull-caudal axis (Figure 12.2).

Occasionally, the rectus abdominis muscles are separated from the midline, creating a diastasis of

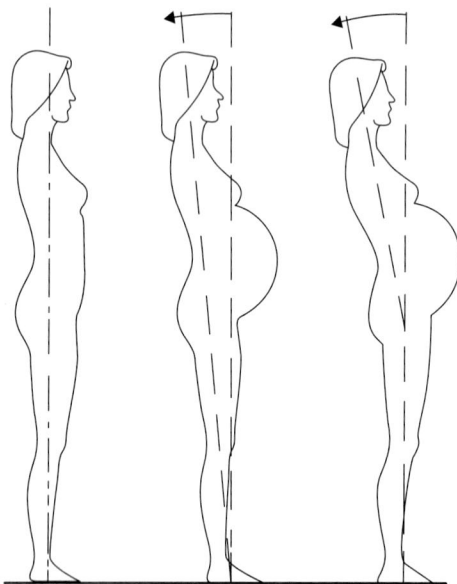

Figure 12.2 Deviation of the center of gravity.
From De Miguel and Sanchez (2001).

variable extension. Sometimes, this phenomenon is so marked that the uterus is only covered by a thin layer of peritoneum, fascia, and skin. The mobility of the sacroiliac joints increases under the control of hormones such as relaxin, and this sometimes causes diffuse pain.

Effect of maternal exercise on pregnant body systems

Pregnancy is a unique process in which nearly all of the body's control systems are modified to maintain both maternal and fetal homeostasis. Since regular physical exercise is today an integral part of the recommendations for a healthy lifestyle, the question remains as to whether exercise may have an adverse effect on pregnancy. In theory, physical exercise during pregnancy should significantly challenge both maternal and fetal well-being due to the conflicting physiological demands of pregnancy and exercise.

The effects of exercise during pregnancy have been extensively explored. However, the low number of well-controlled and adequately powered randomized controlled trials has meant that evidence has been conflicting. Although there is no general consensus regarding the potential long-term risks of or benefits for the offspring of physically active mothers, most studies report that maternal and fetal well-being are not compromised when exercise intensity is light to moderate.

Cardiovascular and hematological response to exercise

The heart rate in pregnant women is significantly higher during exercise compared with nonpregnant women. For stroke volume, similar results have been reported in pregnant and nonpregnant women. Cardiac output increases peaking between 20 and 24 weeks of gestation and thereafter dropping gradually until the end of pregnancy. This decline in the later stages of pregnancy may be due to changes in peripheral vascular resistance and mechanical obstruction of venous return generated by the pressure of the pregnant uterus.

Uteroplacental blood flow response to exercise

Exercise modifies cardiac output by increasing blood flow to active muscle areas at the expense of decreasing flow to other areas such as the uteroplacental unit. Moderate-intensity physical activity causes a reduction in uteroplacental blood flow of ~25%, the magnitude of this reduction being more marked at higher intensities. However, the hypothetical risks posed by exercise blood redistribution are offset by maternal–fetal mechanisms, which ensure maternal and fetal well-being during moderate-intensity aerobic exercise. Particularly, the greatest blood flow reduction occurs in the uterine wall so that the flow of oxygen and nutrients through the placenta is adequate, thus maintaining fetal homeostasis.

In summary, cardiovascular changes caused by moderate-intensity physical activity during pregnancy do not pose a health risk to the mother and fetus in a healthy pregnancy.

Respiratory response to exercise

As stated previously, pulmonary function changes in pregnancy. Hypothetically, exercise causes respiratory modifications that do not occur in nonpregnant women. The effects of moderate intensity physical activity include an increase in most respiratory parameters during pregnancy compared with the non-pregnant state. The respiratory rate tends to increase whether exercise is weight-bearing or not. Most studies have observed a significant increase in minute ventilation and tidal volume, not only at rest, but also during and after exercise. Pregnant women typically show increased ventilation during exertion. Several studies have shown that pregnant women respond with higher minute ventilation than nonpregnant women to the same workload. However, it is important to mention that in pregnancy, maximum oxygen uptake (VO_{2max}.) is achieved at a lower absolute workload.

Thus, respiratory exchange seems to be more difficult in pregnant woman and this problem likely worsens during the course of pregnancy as a result of maternal weight gain and the anatomical changes provoked by the growing uterus.

Hormonal response to exercise

The endocrine changes that occur during pregnancy have profound effects on maternal carbohydrate metabolism, respiratory control, acid–base balance, cardiovascular control, thermoregulation, and other important physiological functions. Indeed, fetal growth and development depend critically on an adequate delivery of oxygenated blood via the uteroplacental circulation, adequate availability of bloodborne substrates (especially glucose), and the maintenance of body temperature within viable limits.

Pregnancy is characterized by a state of reduced peripheral insulin sensitivity and hyperinsulinemia that leads to increased peripheral glucose utilization with decreased glycemia, increased tissue storage of glycogen, and decreased hepatic glucose production. Late in pregnancy, there is a sparing of maternal glucose utilization resulting in reduced maternal levels of glucose and amino acids and ketones, pancreatic islet hypertrophy, and an enhanced insulin response to glucose.

To enable even light-intensity physical activity, there is a continuous uptake of glucose from the blood. Physical activity favors the release of glucose from the liver and of fatty acids from adipose tissue. To maintain steady glucose production, delicate interplay takes place between increased sympathoadrenal and neurohumoral activity, leading to lower plasma insulin and increased concentrations of norepinephrine, epinephrine, cortisol, glucagon, and growth hormone.

During acute exertion of light-moderate intensity, maternal regulatory systems are capable of satisfying both maternal and fetal physiological demands. However, during intense physical activity, particularly if accompanied by nutritional stress, environmental stress or maternal disease, the maternal adaptive reserve might be exceeded.

Effect of maternal exercise on the fetus

Maternal exercise might create a "conflict" between the physiological needs of the growing fetus and those of contracting maternal skeletal muscle. If strenuous exercise is repeated on a chronic basis during occupational work or a physical conditioning program, this could give rise to delayed fetal growth or other developmental abnormalities. Studies conducted in animal models have demonstrated that strenuous maternal exercise can result in a transient reduction in uterine blood flow, the reduced availability of glucose as a metabolic fuel, and increased fetal temperature. In humans, the most common noninvasive method of evaluating fetal well-being is the use of Doppler ultrasound or indirect methods to record fetal heart rate patterns. Several studies have shown that the most common fetal response to maternal moderate-intensity physical activity in healthy pregnant women is an upward drift in fetal heart rate during exercise followed by a gradual recovery to preexercise baseline values in the immediate postexercise period.

Episodes of fetal bradycardia during or following maternal aerobic exercise have also been reported. These findings might be the result of motion artifact caused by maternal pedaling or stepping during cycling or treadmill exercises when fetal heart rate is monitored by Doppler ultrasound. Some authors propose that fetal bradycardia may be the result of transient fetal hypoxia related to venous pooling, reduced venous return, hypotension, and decreased uterine blood flow in the immediate postexercise period.

In summary, occasional episodes of fetal bradycardia during or following maternal exercise have been observed in the fetuses of apparently healthy women and are probably associated with transient moderate fetal hypoxia. The clinical importance of isolated episodes of exercise-induced fetal bradycardia is questionable since such episodes have not been related to an unfavorable pregnancy outcome and might reflect a normal protective autonomic reflex that reduces fetal oxygen utilization.

Effect of maternal exercise on pregnancy outcome

Historically, and largely based more on sociocultural reasons than on scientific evidence, pregnant women have been encouraged to reduce their physical activity and stop working during pregnancy because of a perceived increased risk of problems, such as early pregnancy loss or a reduced gestational age.

In recent years, numerous studies, especially clinical trials, have addressed issues concerning maternal exercise and its potential effects on (maternal and fetal) pregnancy outcome. The results of many studies over the last decade have indicated few or no negative effects of physical activity on the outcome of a healthy pregnancy if the physical activity is of moderate intensity. However, if the intensity of exercise regularly exceeds the threshold of "moderate" for long periods of pregnancy, pregnancy outcome may be compromised, as demonstrated in several animal studies.

Most of the maternal factors examined have revealed no association between physical activity and an adverse pregnancy outcome for the mother. Among the more commonly examined variables, we find overall maternal weight gain, gestational age, or type of delivery.

The most commonly assessed factors in newborns have been birth weight, size, and the Apgar score.

Overall maternal weight gain during pregnancy

The Institute of Medicine & National Research Council (Washington, USA, 2009) recommends that normal-weight women should gain an extra weight between 11.4 and 15.9 kg during pregnancy, while overweight pregnant women should gain an extra weight between 6.8 and 11.4 kg. Weight gains within these guidelines are associated with healthy fetal and maternal outcomes while weight gains below these goals are linked to a low infant birth-weight and higher weight gains to fetal macrosomia.

Excessive maternal weight gain especially has been related to a number of adverse outcomes during and after pregnancy, such as gestational diabetes, preeclampsia, cesarean delivery, and a high birthweight for gestational age, as well as an increased risk of childhood obesity.

In addition, over 60% of overweight women gain more than the recommended weight during pregnancy. Also, as gestational weight gain is directly associated with maternal weight retained during the postpartum period and with adiposity in childhood and early adulthood, excess gestational weight gain could accelerate the obesity epidemic.

Current recommendations are that pregnant women should undertake moderate-intensity exercise for 30 minutes or more on most, if not all, days of the week. In general, women tend to be insufficiently active during pregnancy and women who have a high prepregnancy BMI are even less likely to be physically active.

Indeed, pregnancy is a critical period in the life of a women and this means she may be more receptive to behavior change interventions. Encouraging physical activity is a key component of weight control interventions as it has beneficial effects on glucose metabolism. It has also been suggested that physical activity may improve pregnancy outcome independently of weight.

Several studies have examined the effect of moderate-intensity aerobic exercise on maternal weight in pregnancy, and most have identified a beneficial effect, that is, attenuation of excessive weight gain even in previously obese women.

Gestational age

Throughout history, the possibility of a reduced gestational age has been one of the main reasons for denying women access to regular exercise programs during pregnancy. Thus, advice about the type, duration, and intensity of exercise during pregnancy has been based more on cultural and moral issues than on scientific evidence.

Studies that have examined the influence of moderate regular exercise programs during pregnancy have found no gestational age alterations in healthy pregnant women. However, many researchers warn of the risk of preterm delivery associated with high-intensity exercise, especially in late pregnancy due mainly to elevated norepinephrine levels in maternal blood flow causing early uterine contractions.

Type of delivery

While many studies have focused on maternal outcomes such as total weight gain and gestational age, less data are available on the association between physical activity during pregnancy and the type of delivery. A few studies showed that, in previously well-conditioned women, continuation of their exercise regimens (aerobics or running) during the second half of pregnancy had a beneficial effect on the course and outcome of labor (*i.e.*, lower incidence of abdominal and normal [vaginal] operative delivery). This is in agreement with prospective data on previously sedentary nulliparous women that indicate that regular participation in aerobic exercise during the first two trimesters of pregnancy can lower the risk of a cesarean delivery.

The results of a recent clinical trial also revealed a lower percentage of Cesarean sections in active women compared with those who remained inactive during pregnancy

Effects on the fetus/newborn

Apgar score, weight, and body size at birth is a marker of the intrauterine environment. Fetal adaptation to an adverse intrauterine environment involves the reprogramming of metabolic pathways that might predispose the newborn to cardiovascular disease in later life. This adverse environment can modify gene expression profiles leading to physiological phenotypes associated with a greater risk of morbidity and mortality. Low-birthweight newborns show an increased risk of perinatal as well as adult morbidity and mortality, whereas high-birthweight newborns have an increased risk of several complications, such as shoulder dystocia, operative delivery, and birth canal lacerations. A high birthweight has been also associated with an increased risk during adulthood of type 2 diabetes and some types of cancer.

Studies examining the effects of exercise on the overall health of the fetus and newborn have revealed that neonatal outcome does not differ significantly in women who exercise during pregnancy and sedentary women. This means that, from a global perspective, exercise during pregnancy has no adverse effects on the health of the fetus or newborn.

Birthweight is the most frequently assessed factor because of the effect that this variable has on a child's later life. A recent clinical trial has shown that women who stay active during pregnancy are less likely to deliver macrosomic babies.

Thus, maternal exercise during pregnancy could prevent fetal macrosomia and other neonatal complications. Accordingly, health care professionals should focus on improving the well-being of mother and fetus/new born by recommending regular programs of moderate physical exercise during pregnancy.

Recommendations on exercise during pregnancy and the postpartum

Exercise type

Aerobic: low impact activities are recommended such as walking, trekking, dancing, swimming, and biking.

Strength training: 1 set of 12 repetitions of exercises targeting major muscle groups are recommended in the form of circuit training. Strength exercise should be performed at controlled speeds and with low weights. The use of elastic bands can also be used.

Intensity

Intensity should fall within the light-to-moderate range, depending on the fitness level of the women. Heart rate should be between 60% and 70% of maximum heart rate [209 − (0.73 × age)], or 4 to 8 METs. However, heart rate might not be a good physiological indicator of intensity in this population so we suggest the use of easier tools. Such tools include an effort perception scale, with scores from 0 to 10, where sitting is assigned 0 and sprinting 10. According to this scale, a light intensity of exercise would correspond to a score of 0–2, light to moderate intensity to one of 4–5, and moderate to vigorous intensity to one of 5–6.

In women with little or no previous experience with exercising, the talk test could be used to assess exercise intensity.

Duration

Pregnant women should engage in 150 minutes/week of light to moderate intensity aerobic exercise spread across the week: ideally, 30 minutes/day for at least 5 days/week. Bouts of about 10 minutes can also be performed. For previously sedentary pregnant women, a lighter exercise regimen might also induce health benefits.

It is not advisable to perform exercise for periods longer than 60 minutes. Nevertheless, overall exercise duration will vary much depend on exercise intensity, fitness level, and on the duration of resting periods.

Frequency

Physical activity should be carried out at least 5 days/week. It is likely that sedentary women will gain benefits from 3 days of physical activity per week. The recommended frequency of many exercise programs for pregnant women is 3 days/week, such that at least a further 2 days of physical activity should be added.

Special considerations
• Physical activity is recommended from the first trimester of pregnancy. Light-intensity activities such as walking, biking, or swimming are ideal. Increase both the time and intensity gradually.
• Before starting an exercise session, a light short warm-up of about 5–10 minutes is needed. Similarly, each exercise session should end with a cooling-down period of 5–10 minutes consisting of relaxing and stretching activities.
• Hydration: We recommend drinking at least 33 mL of water every 30 minutes.
• Physical activity is also recommended for pregnant women with gestational diabetes, obesity, or hypertension.
• Elite athletes will experience the same physiological limitations as those who are not athletes, and will be able to continue with their training regimen as long as they are able to keep up the normal time and intensity. It is recommended to gradually decrease both exercise time and intensity as pregnancy ensues. Competitive-related stress should be avoided.

• Physically active pregnant women with a history of premature labor should reduce exercise duration and intensity.

• Physical activity does not affect breast-feeding.

• In the case of a scheduled cesarean delivery, it is recommended to gradually start performing physical activity in the 6th week of pregnancy.

Things to avoid

• High-risk activities such as snorkeling, contact sports, or jumps.

• Activities carrying a high risk of falling such as skiing or skating, or activities placing high demands on abdominal muscles. The type of exercise undertaken will, however, largely depend on the mother's level of experience.

• Valsalva maneuver.

• Isometric strength training involving major muscle groups.

• Standing still for long periods of time.

• Physical activity at high altitude (>2500–3000 m), especially if the mother is not acclimatized.

• Very hot temperatures and high humidity.

Contraindications for aerobic exercise

• Hemodynamically significant heart disease;

• restrictive lung disease;

• incompetent cervix/cervical cerclage;

• multiple gestation at risk for premature labor;

• persistent second- or third-trimester bleeding;

• placenta previa after 26 weeks of gestation;

• premature labor during the current pregnancy;

• ruptured membranes; and

• preeclampsia/pregnancy-induced hypertension.

Relative contraindications for aerobic exercise

• Severe anemia;

• nonassessed maternal cardiac arrhythmia;

• chronic bronchitis;

• poorly controlled type 1 diabetes;

• extreme morbid obesity;

• extreme underweight (BMI <12);

• history of extremely sedentary lifestyle;

• intrauterine growth restriction in current pregnancy;

• poorly controlled hypertension;

• orthopedic limitations;

• poorly controlled seizure disorder;

• poorly controlled hyperthyroidism; and

• heavy smoker.

Signs indicating exercise should be terminated while pregnant

• Vaginal bleeding;

• dyspnea prior to exertion;

• dizziness;

• headache;

• chest pain;

• muscle weakness;

• calf pain or swelling (need to rule out thrombophlebitis);

• preterm labor;

• diminished fetal movement; and

• amniotic fluid leakage.

Examples of how to meet physical activity recommendations

For those who are sedentary

• Light-moderate intensity walking for 10 minutes, 1–2 times/day, 2–3 days/week combined with a resistance training circuit with elastic bands of about 10 minutes, 1–2 days/week.

• Biking 10–15 minutes, 1–2 times/day, 2–3 days/week, combined with a resistance training circuit with elastic bands of about 10 minutes, 1–2 days/week.

• Dancing 2 days/week, and walking around 30 minutes, 3 days/week.

• 30 minutes of water activities 2 days/week, 30 minutes biking 2 days/week combined with a resistance training circuit with elastic bands of about 10 minutes, 1–2 days/week, trekking.

For those who are physically active

• Brisk walking 50–60 minutes, 5 days/week combined with a resistance training circuit with elastic bands of about 10–20 minutes, 1–2 days/week.

• Biking 30–40 minutes, 5 days/week combined with a resistance training circuit with elastic bands of about 10–20 minutes, 1–2 days/week.

• Swimming 45 minutes, 3 days/week, brisk walking 45 minutes, 3 days/week combined with a resistance training circuit with elastic bands of about 10–20 minutes, 1–2 days/week.

• Dancing 45 minutes, 3 days/week, and brisk walking.

• Special attention should be paid to the musculature of the pelvic floor, independently of the type of labor.

• Women can initiate their normal physical activity (low impact) within 15–20 days of delivery in the case of normal labor, within 25–30 days in the case of instrumental labor with episiotomy, or within 35–45 days in the case of cesarean delivery.

• Activities of a certain impact are not recommended, with the exception of jogging 20–25 days after a delivery with no complications, or 35–40 days after an instrumental labor with episiotomy and with gynecologist approval.

Special recommendations for the post-partum period

Exercise program examples for sedentary pregnant women

Type	Activity	Intensity (0–10)	METs	Duration (min)	Times per day	Times per week
Aerobic	Slow walking	Light (2–3)	2–4	10	1–3	2–3
Aerobic	Walking	Light-moderate (3–4)	2–6	10–15	1–2	2–3
Aerobic	Treadmill walking	Light: 2–3 km/h (2–3)	2–4	10–15	1–2	2–3
		Moderate: 5 km/h (3–5)	4–6	10–15	1–2	2–3
Aerobic	Biking	Light (2–3)	2–4	10	1–3	2–3
		Light-moderate (3–4)	2–6	10–15	1–2	2–3
Aerobic and strength	Water activities	Light (2–3)	2–4	30	1	2–3
		Light-moderate (3–4)	4–6	30	1	2–3
Aerobic	Dancing	Light-moderate (3–4)	2–6	30	1	2–3
Strength	Resistance training	Light (2–3)	2–4	8–10	1	1–2
Aerobic	Yoga, Tai-chi	Light (2–3)	2–4	30	1	2–3

Exercise program examples for physically active pregnant women

Type	Activity	Intensity (0–10)	METs	Duration (min)	Times per day	Times per week
Aerobic	Walking	Moderate (4–5)	4–6	30–40	1	5–6
Aerobic	Brisk walking	Moderate-vigorous (5–6)	4–8	30	1	5–6
	Treadmill waking	Moderate: 4–5 km/h	4–6	15	2	5–6
Aerobic		Moderate-vigorous: 5–6 km/h	4–8	10–15	1–2	5–6
Aerobic	Static biking	Moderate-vigorous (5–6)	4–8	15–20	1–2	2–3
Aerobic and strength	"Aquagym"	Moderate (4–5)	4–6	40–50	1	2–3
		Moderate-vigorous (5–6)	4–7	30–40	1	2–3
Aerobic and strength	Dancing/aerobic	Moderate-vigorous (5–6)	4–8	30–40	1	2–3
Strength	Resistance training	Moderate (4–5)	4–6	10–20	1	2
Aerobic	Yoga, Tai-chi	Light-moderate (3–4)	2–6	30	1	2–3

It is recommended to combine different types of activity.

Physical activity recommendations during pregnancy and the postpartum

- Avoid a sedentary lifestyle
- Women with a pregestational sedentary lifestyle should engage in at least 150 minutes of moderate-intensity aerobic exercise over the week, that is, at least 30 minutes/day. Light-intensity strength training should be performed 1–2 times/week.
- Women with a pregestational active lifestyle should continue with their normal exercise regimen bearing in mind that both duration and intensity should not be high.

These recommendations should be added to a person's routine daily life activities.

Recommended reading

American College of Obstetricians and Gynecologists. (2002) Exercise during pregnancy and the postpartum period. Committee Opinion No 267. Washington, DC. *Obstet Gynecol*, 99, 171–173.

Artal R, Wiswell R, and Drinkwater B. (1991) *Exercise in Pregnancy* (2nd edn). Williams and Wilkins, Baltimore, MD.

Barakat R, Lucia A, and Ruiz J. (2009) Resistance exercise training during pregnancy and newborn's birth size: a randomised controlled trial. *Int J Obes (Lond)*, 33(9), 1048–1057.

Barakat R, Ruiz JR, Stirling JR, Zakynthinaki M, and Lucia A. (2009) Type of delivery is not affected by light resistance and toning exercise training during pregnancy: a randomized controlled trial. *Am J Obstet Gynecol*, 201(6), 590.

De Miguel J, Sanchez M. (2001) Physiological changes and maternal adaptation during pregnancy. In: E. Fabre Gonzalez (ed), *Working Group on Assistance to normal pregnancy: Section of Perinatal Medicine*. Chapter 4. Spanish Society of Gynaecology and Obstetrics. Manual of assistance to normal pregnancy (2nd edn). Zaragoza, Spain.

Mottola M and Wolfe L. (2000) The pregnant athlete. In: B Drinkwater (ed), *Woman in Sport*. Blackwell Science.

Ruiz J, Pelaez M, Perales M, *et al.* (2013) Supervised exercise-based intervention to prevent excessive gestational weight gain: a randomised controlled trial. *Mayo Clin Proc*, 88(12), 1388–1397.

Wolfe L, Brenner I, and Mottola M. (1994) Maternal exercise, fetal well-being and pregnancy outcome. *Exerc Sport Sci Rev*, 22, 145–194.

Wolfe LA, Ohtake P, Mottola M, and McGrath MJ. (1989) Physiological interactions between pregnancy and aerobic exercise, *Exerc Sport Sci Rev*, 17, 295–351.

Chapter 13
The paralympic female athlete

Cheri A. Blauwet

Department of Physical Medicine and Rehabilitation, Spaulding Rehabilitation Hospital/Brigham and Women's Hospital, Harvard Medical School, Boston, MA, USA

Introduction and background

Since the inception of the Paralympic Movement, the unique needs of female Paralympic athletes have remained a growing area of focus and attention. The Paralympic Movement is said to have originated in Stoke Mandeville, England in 1948. At that time, a total of 16 athletes (14 men, 2 women) competed in the sport of archery, with a predominant focus on the use of sport as a proactive tool for rehabilitation and physical fitness. The first modern Paralympic Games took place in 1960 in Rome, Italy, at which time Paralympic athletes competed in the same city, utilizing the same venues as their Olympic counterparts. With the growth of the Games and an expansion in the number of sports included on the Paralympic schedule, increasing numbers of female athletes have become involved in Paralympic sports (Figure 13.1). Concurrently, there has been a progressive shift of the Games from a tool for medical rehabilitation to the elite, competitive sporting event it is today. At the most recent London 2012 Paralympic Games, 1501 female athletes competed, representing 35% of the total athlete count and a 10% proportional increase from the

Sydney 2000 Paralympic Games only 12 years prior (Figure 13.1). Currently, 18 of the total 20 sports on the summer Paralympic schedule include female competitors (Figure 13.2). Additionally, via Paralympic sport, women with varied categories of impairment are offered the opportunity to compete on the world's stage. These include women with spinal cord injury (SCI), spina bifida, cerebral palsy, achondroplasia, visual impairment, and limb loss, among others. Ongoing advocacy initiatives remain focused on expanding these opportunities and increasing the representation of female Paralympic athletes globally.

As the role of women in Paralympic sport grows, the unique health needs of female athletes with disabilities have come to the forefront as an area of study and professional focus for sports medicine practitioners. The vast majority of the health and medical needs of women with disabilities remain similar to their able-bodied counterparts. In this way, team physicians, athletic trainers, and allied health professionals are qualified to provide medical care to athletes with a disability, whether in a one-on-one clinical setting or via team or mass participation event coverage. Issues of sports-related injury and illness, bone health, genitourinary function, and autonomic control do in fact vary for female athletes with a disability. For these topics, this chapter will provide an overview as to the needs of this specific population. Additionally, the sociopolitical context of female athlete participation in Paralympic sport will be briefly discussed.

The Female Athlete, First Edition. Edited by Margo L. Mountjoy.
© 2015 International Olympic Committee. Published 2015 by John Wiley & Sons, Inc.

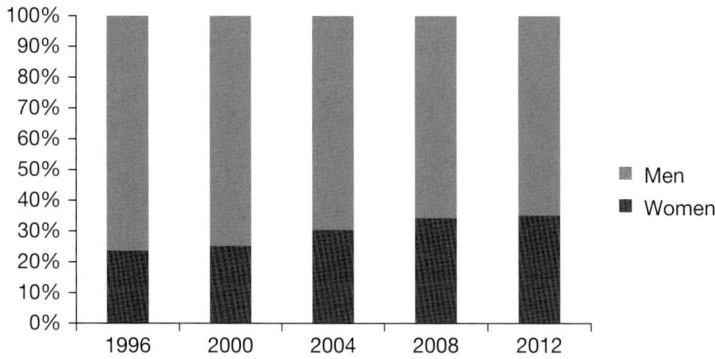

Figure 13.1 Gender participation by proportion at the summer paralympic games, 1996–2012 (Courtesy of the International Paralympic Committee).

Injury and illness prevention

In Paralympic sport, the incidence and characteristics of both injury and illness are disability and sport specific. An increased awareness of the quantity and type of injuries that athletes may incur while in major international competition enables team medical staff to more adequately prepare for event coverage and anticipate the needs of female Paralympic athletes. In 2002, the Paralympic Injury Surveillance Study (ISS) was initiated at the winter Paralympic Games in Salt Lake City as a means of providing longitudinal tracking of injuries as well as for monitoring injury prevention strategies. Following successful implementation of the Paralympic ISS during the 2002, 2006, and 2010 Winter

Games, the project was expanded at the London 2012 Summer Games to include tracking of both sports-related injuries and also medical illnesses.

With few exceptions, the incidence of injury and medical illness in Paralympic sport are similar when comparing male and female athletes. For example, at the Vancouver 2010 Winter Paralympic Games, 33 injuries were recorded among 124 female athletes (incidence proportion = 26.6%), while 87 injuries were recorded among 381 male athletes (incidence proportion = 22.8%) (Webborn *et al.*, 2012). There was no significant difference in the incidence proportion (IP) of injury based on sex. For those sports in which female athletes competed, alpine skiing showed the highest IP of injury at 21.6%, although it remains unknown if this varied for male versus female athletes.

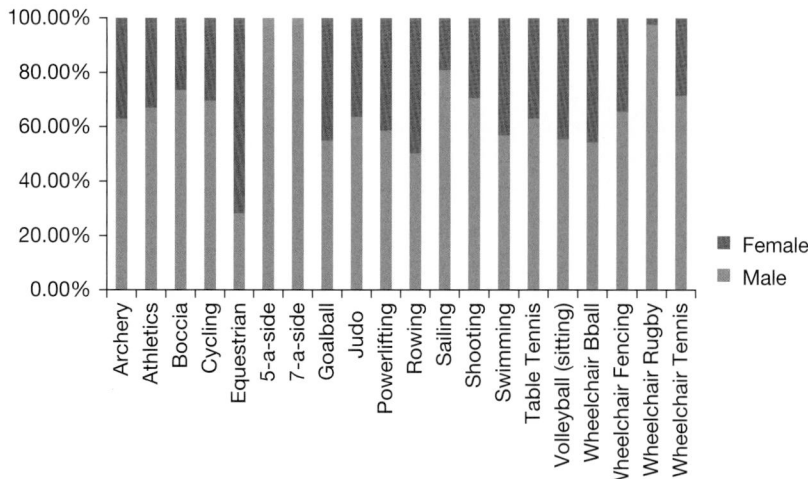

Figure 13.2 Gender participation by sport at the London 2012 Paralympic Games (note: athletics is the international nomenclature for track and field) (Courtesy of the International Paralympic Committee).

Data regarding injury and medical illness in summer Paralympic sport reveals similar trends when comparing male and female athletes. With expansion of the Paralympic Injury and Illness Surveillance Study to the London 2012 Summer Paralympic Games, athlete exposure data was also collected, thus allowing for the calculation of incidence rate (IR) of injury, defined as injuries per 1000 athlete days. Overall, this revealed 196 injuries in 1218 female athletes, yielding an IR of 11.5 injuries per 1000 athlete days (95% CI 9.9–13.2) (Willick *et al.*, 2013). Similarly, 437 injuries in 2347 male athletes were recorded, yielding an IR of 13.3 injuries per 1000 athlete days (95% CI 12.1–14.6). For the total Games period, there was no significant difference in the IR of injury in female versus male athletes. Of note, female athletes did experience a higher IR of injury in the precompetition period (IR = 16.7, 95% CI 12.8–21.4) when compared to the competition period (IR = 10.1, 95% CI 8.4–11.9). This may be due to poor health care access for many female Paralympains in their home nations, thus leading athletes to seek care for both acute and chronic injuries upon first arrival to the Games and prior to the start of competition. Overall, for both male and female Paralympic athletes, the shoulder was the most commonly injured anatomical region, representing 17.7% of all injuries over the total study period. Given these findings, it can be extrapolated that medical professionals covering major Paralympic events (assuming a team size of 100 athletes over a 10-day period) should expect to see approximately 11–12 injuries in female athletes, with a predominance of upper extremity involvement.

Regarding rates of medical illness at the summer 2012 Paralympic Games, overall 251 illnesses in 1218 female athletes were recorded, yielding an IR of 14.4 (95% CI 12.6–16.3) (Schwellnus *et al.*, 2013). In comparison, 2347 male athletes experienced 424 illnesses yielding an IR of 12.5 (95% CI 11.4–13.8). There was no significant difference between male and female athletes with respect to the IR of illness. For female athletes, the sports of athletics (track and field), archery, and equestrian revealed the highest incidence rate of illness. In these sports as well as several others, greater than 20% of female athletes experienced illness during the Summer Paralympic Games. Illnesses most commonly involved the respiratory system followed by the skin and subcutaneous tissue. Overall, these findings can be extrapolated to conclude that medical professionals covering major Paralympic events (again, assuming a team size of 100 athletes over a 10-day period) should plan to see approximately 14–15 medical illnesses in female athletes, with a predominance of these involving the respiratory system (Figure 13.3).

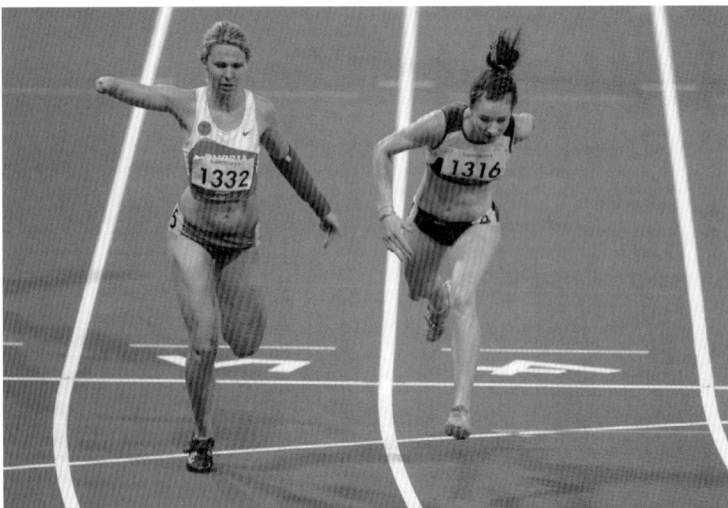

Figure 13.3 Female summer Paralympic athletes show high incidence rates of illness in the sports of athletics, archery, and equestrian (Photo courtesy of Mr Herman Verwey).

Bone health

Issues of bone health remain of utmost importance for injury prevention strategies and to optimize sports performance. For nonambulatory female Paralympic athletes, the effects of decreased bone mineral density due to a low weight-bearing status may be compounded by the more commonly observed age-related changes and/or the female athlete triad. For these athletes, attention must be given to the optimization of bone health and the prevention of fracture during sports competition.

Female athletes with a disability may experience a decrease in weight bearing status via several distinct mechanisms. For some athletes this may occur acutely, as in the case of adult onset neurologic disability such as SCI. In these athletes, a rapid decrease in trabecular bone mineral content below the level of neurologic injury may occur at a rate of up to 4% per month post injury, with an estimated 40% reduction in bone mineral density by several years post injury (Dauty et al., 2000). Additionally, trabecular bone loss in postmenopausal women with complete SCI may be greater than in ambulatory postmenopausal women (Slade et al., 2005). For female athletes with a disability that has been present from a young age such as cerebral palsy, bone health may depend on the degree of weight bearing longitudinally over time. Although the relative decrease in bone mineral content for these athletes is less dramatic than in those with a new onset acute neurologic injury, overall bone mineral density is frequently reduced when compared to their age-matched peers.

In cases of acute sports-related trauma in nonambulatory female athletes, sports medicine professionals must maintain a high index of suspicion for fracture. For example, in females with SCI, the most common sites for lower extremity fracture include the distal femur and proximal tibia (Vestergaard et al., 1998). Further complicating the picture, these athletes will frequently have decreased lower extremity sensation and thus a lower likelihood of reporting acute pain secondary to fracture. In these circumstances, a thorough physical exam of the lower extremities should be accompanied by radiologic imaging of any area deemed particularly concerning, with follow-up to monitor for the development of swelling, ecchymosis, or limb deformity. Distal pulses should also be monitored to rule out vascular compromise. These recommendations are most pertinent in sports that incur the risk of high-speed trauma, such as alpine skiing, wheelchair racing, and handcycling, although low-velocity trauma may also lead to fracture. Nondisplaced fractures of osteoporotic bone can easily be missed on plain radiographs; therefore clinicians should have a low threshold for proceeding with advanced imaging if a fracture is suspected.

Longitudinally, care should be taken to optimize bone health in female athletes with a disability as a focus of sports injury prevention. Vitamin D levels may be monitored to ensure these remain in the normal range, with appropriate repletion as necessary for athletes with levels <30 ng/mL. In athletes for whom dietary availability of calcium may be low, supplementation is advised. The use of bisphosphonates remains controversial and should be reserved for female athletes who are not of child-bearing age, with low bone mineral density confirmed via dual energy X-ray absorptiometry (DEXA) in consultation with a bone-health specialist. For the population of female athletes with a disability who are less than 50 years of age, calculation of a Z-score is the most appropriate measure of bone mineral density. Scores less than two standard deviations below age-matched normal values constitute osteoporosis that may increase the risk of fracture (Figure 13.4).

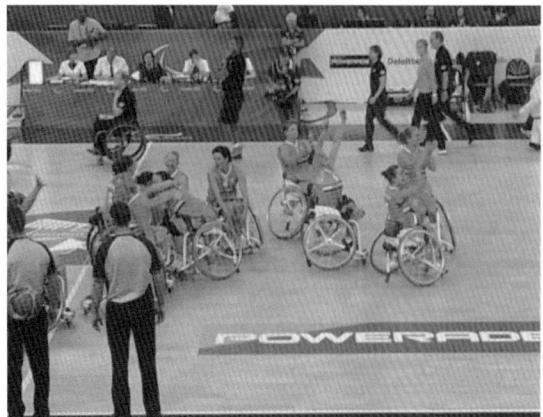

Figure 13.4 Nonambulatory female Paralympic athletes must be aware of the importance of optimizing bone health (Photo courtesy Dr Stuart Willick).

Ultimately, maintaining a safe sporting environment remains the most effective preventative mechanism to minimize fracture risk within this unique population. Female athletes with a disability must be educated regarding the importance of bone health and fracture risk with low-velocity trauma, while ensuring a safe competition environment to minimize injury.

Bowel and bladder considerations

Among female athletes with a disability, bowel and bladder management remains of great importance in promoting athlete health and optimal sports performance. In addition to the potential effects of stress incontinence and pelvic floor dysfunction, many female athletes with a disability may also experience increased difficulty in maintaining optimal genitourinary and gastrointestinal health. Neurogenic bowel and bladder dysfunction occur secondary to a loss of central neurologic control of bowel and bladder emptying. An awareness of this phenomenon is essential for medical personnel working with female athletes with a disability at all sport participation levels from developmental to elite.

Voluntary bowel and bladder function are controlled by a complex interplay between central and peripheral neurologic control centers, which in optimal circumstances enable continence at socially appropriate times. In Paralympic athletes with neurologic injuries such as SCI, spina bifida, and cerebral palsy, among others, these control centers may be impaired, thus requiring the athletes to utilize alternative means for bladder emptying and bowel evacuation.

As related to genitourinary function, neurogenic bladder may result from injury to the cerebral cortex or pontine micturition center (e.g., in athletes who have experienced a stroke or cerebral palsy), the ascending/descending spinal cord tracts or the spinal cord sacral micturition center (e.g., SCI or spina bifida), or the sacral nerve roots themselves (e.g., SCI, cauda equina type). Dysfunction in various regions of this complex neurologic pathway will result in different subtypes of neurogenic bladder, a discussion of which is beyond the scope of this chapter. In sum, athletes will typically experience either an overactive, spastic bladder, or a flaccid bladder with difficulty emptying. For both conditions, female athletes will typically employ an intermittent self-catheterization protocol for predictable emptying in appropriate settings. Alternatively, for female athletes with upper extremity impairments resulting in difficulty with toilet transfers and/or decreased hand dexterity, bladder emptying may be accomplished by the use of an indwelling suprapubic or urethral catheter. This option enables female athletes to void in a hygienic fashion without having to transfer into or out of a wheelchair.

Medications may be utilized to assist with bladder management in female athletes. For the treatment of overactive, spastic bladder, anticholinergic agents such as oxybutynin are frequently prescribed to inhibit spastic activity of the detrusor muscle, thus improving bladder storage capacity. For female athletes with a flaccid, underactive bladder, self-catheterization remains the mainstay of treatment to ensure complete bladder emptying. Of note, for antidoping purposes, female athletes should be educated regarding the importance of having a sterile urinary catheter available for sample collection and to avoid potential contamination. Additionally, many female athletes will purposefully become dehydrated during long-haul international travel due to concern for difficulty accessing the lavatory or inaccessible restroom facilities. In this circumstance, it is advised that female athletes take care to stay well hydrated for several days prior and several days after the travel period in order to ensure adequate hydration at the time of training and competition.

For female athletes with neurogenic bladder, the incidence of urinary tract infection (UTI) is higher than for those who do not have bladder dysfunction. For this reason, UTI should be suspected in any female athlete who meets all of the following criteria: (1) the presence of bacteria in the urine, (2) the presence of white blood cells in the urine (pyuria), and (3) the onset of new symptoms (Linsenmeyer et al., 2010). Symptoms may include dysuria, urinary frequency, cloudy urine, or foul-smelling urine. For athletes with decreased genitourinary sensation, however, symptoms such as fatigue, malaise, increased spasticity, or low-grade fever may be indicative of UTI in the absence of other classic symptoms. If infection is suspected, appropriate antibiotic treatment should be initiated immediately to prevent more significant illness and thus a detrimental impact on sports performance.

For purposes of promoting optimal bowel management, many female athletes will employ what is termed a "bowel program" in order to achieve a bowel movement at a time that is convenient for daily life activities and optimal sports performance. Similar to what has been noted for the bladder, colonic neurologic pathways are controlled via both central and peripheral mechanisms. Neurogenic bowel may result from injury to the cerebral cortex, the ascending/descending spinal cord tracts, the spinal cord sacral control center, or the sacral nerve roots. Additionally, injury to the enteric nervous system carrying autonomic fibers (Meissner's and Auerbach's plexus within the colonic submucosa and muscularis externa, respectively) may result in decreased involuntary peristalsis and thus decreased colonic motility and forward movement of stool through the gastrointestinal tract. Most typically, female athletes will optimize their routine for planned colonic emptying with the use of oral cathartic agents such as docusate, senokot, and polyethylene glycol, or rectal agents such as bisacodyl or glycerin suppositories.

Female athletes with a disability will often have tremendous insight into their own bowel and bladder management, thus promoting maximal functional independence and optimizing sport performance. As sports medicine professionals, our primary role in this setting is to provide support to ensure the availability of accessible facilities and to assist with medication or supply management in the event that a change in routine is necessary. Ultimately, each female athlete should remain autonomous in her preferred methods of optimizing bowel and bladder management. For those female athletes requiring additional advice regarding the establishment of a continent bowel or bladder program, referral to a specialist in physical medicine and rehabilitation or urology is recommended.

Autonomic dysreflexia and female paralympic athletes

Autonomic dysreflexia (AD), a reflex syndrome experienced by athletes with an SCI at or above the level of T6, is a condition unique to Paralympic sport. In these athletes, the experience of a noxious stimulus below the level of neurologic injury often results in an uncontrolled sympathetic response with massive release of noradrenaline (and, to a smaller degree, adrenaline). When this occurs, given the presence of an SCI, the brain cannot provide central descending inhibitory control to levels of the sympathetic chain below the level of injury, and the athlete is left in an acute hyperadrenergic state until the noxious stimulus is removed. AD may result in signs and symptoms such as acute hypertension, headache, diaphoresis, piloerection, and feelings of aggression or anxiety. Given the acute hypertensive crisis often seen with a dysreflexic response, AD is considered a medical emergency for individuals with SCI.

AD most frequently occurs as the result of visceral distension, such as with bladder overfilling or constipation. Other sources of noxious stimuli may also lead to a dysreflexic response, such as the lower extremities being "strapped in" too tight in an athletic wheelchair, skin breakdown below the level of neurologic injury, or other stimulus which may cause pain to an insensate area of the body. In women with SCI, mild dysreflexia may be elicited during times of premenstrual cramping. Additionally, the nature of sport competition itself may lead to AD, such as with on-court collisions in the sport of wheelchair rugby. For this reason, it is essential for sports medicine professionals to be aware of the signs and symptoms of AD. If a dysreflexic response occurs, the inciting noxious stimulus must be removed in order to relieve symptoms. This is most frequently accomplished by emptying the bladder. If an athlete experiences AD during or just prior to competition, he or she must be taken out of the play until the episode is resolved.

In recent years, the prohibited method of "boosting," defined as the intentional induction of AD for performance enhancement purposes, has come under increased scrutiny (Blauwet et al., 2013). In athletes susceptible to AD the normal cardiovascular response to exercise is typically reduced given impaired sympathetic activation (Krassioukov, 2012). By purposefully inducing AD, these athletes are able to overcome their own inherent physiologic limitations to exercise, thus leading to improved sports performance. Studies specific to the sport of wheelchair racing have shown AD to be an effective means of improving race time by as much as 10% (Burnham et al,, 1994). In order to promote fair play and ensure athlete safety, boosting is strictly banned by the International Paralympic Committee (IPC), and recent action has been taken in an attempt to deter its practice. Under IPC rules, both male and female athletes with SCI at or above the level of T6 are subject to random blood pressure screening prior to competition (IPC, 2013). If the systolic blood pressure is found to be dangerously elevated, the athlete may be disqualified from competition due to the presence of boosting and to ensure his or her safety and fitness to compete.

Public health implications of disability sport and the female athlete

As the participation of women with disabilities in competitive sport grows, so does our understanding of the ongoing disparities in access to sport and physical activity opportunities for this population at all levels, from developmental to elite. In this setting, the concept of "double discrimination" is often considered. Double discrimination is the compounded systemic exclusion that women with disabilities may encounter due to both gender and disability-related discrimination. In the context of sport, it remains the case that distinct effort must be made to promote the participation of women with disabilities in both developed as well as resource-poor settings. In addition to the use of sport to enhance opportunities for women with disabilities, the conceptualization of sport, physical activity, and exercise as a critical component of health maintenance and the prevention of

noncommunicable disease remains of the utmost importance.

Protecting the rights of female athletes with a disability also remains a focus of ongoing advocacy initiatives. In both sport- and nonsport-based settings, it is commonly accepted that women with disabilities are at increased risk of experiencing sexual harassment and abuse. Additionally, due to ongoing societal stigma, women with disabilities are more often hidden within the community. Frequently, grassroots sports opportunities can be utilized as a catalyst for the increased socialization of women with disabilities, as well as a tool to improve stature and visibility. Reflecting this, the recently drafted United Nations Convention on the Rights of Persons with Disabilities (CRPD) is inclusive of Article 30, the "Right to Participation in Cultural Life, Recreation, Leisure and Sport" (United Nations, 2006).

Despite these efforts, barriers for participation of women with disabilities in physical activity and sport frequently persist. Additionally, recruitment of female Paralympians remains a significant challenge in many world regions. At an elite level, in comparison to the Olympic Games, the proportion of female athlete participation in the Paralympic Games lags by approximately 10% (Figure 13.5). Given the estimated global prevalence of disability to be at or around 20% of the total population, this disparity can be attributed to a lack of access to sport rather than an insufficient number of potential participants.

To address these ongoing disparities, in 2000 the IPC Women in Sport Committee was formed for the purpose of promoting the representation and voice of female Paralympians within the movement. Ongoing initiatives include efforts to increase the number of female Paralympians in leadership positions, increase the proportion of female athletes competing in the Games, and to ensure mentorship opportunities for young female Paralympic athletes through the "WoMentoring" program (Tileman, 2013). Additionally, specific focus has been given to the expansion of grassroots opportunities for women with disabilities to become involved in sport as a tool for health, fitness, and increased community visibility. For example, the National

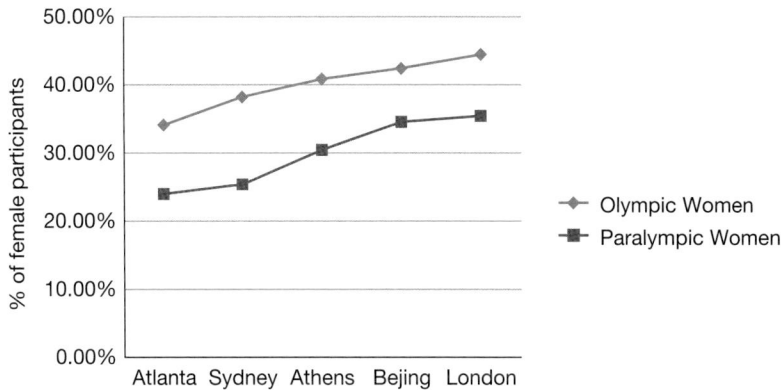

Figure 13.5 Trends in female participation in the Paralympic Games in comparison to the Olympic Games (Courtesy of the International Paralympic Committee).

Paralympic Committee of Rwanda has preferentially increased the number of female athletes on their developmental national team through the expansion of the sport of sitting volleyball, in which athletes with limb loss may compete without the need for expensive equipment (C. Nzeyimana, personal communication). Additionally, the recent acquisition of several racing wheelchairs from the international nongovernmental organization, Motivation, in partnership with the IPC Agitos Foundation, will be allocated preferentially to women in order to promote participation.

Conclusion

Although the majority of health and medical needs of female athletes with an impairment do not vary on the basis of disability; several key factors should be taken into consideration to optimize athlete health and sports performance. A general knowledge of injury prevention, bone health, bowel and bladder management, and the prevention of AD is essential for sports medicine professionals responsible for the care of female athletes with a disability. Additionally, ongoing efforts to promote and enhance the competitive opportunities for this athlete population must be emphasized to ensure access and equality of opportunity at both developmental and elite levels of sport into the future.

Acknowledgments

The author wishes to thank several colleagues who were instrumental in the development and review of this chapter, namely Dr Maria Reese, Dr Ellen Casey, Dr Stuart Willick, Dr Peter van de Vliet, Dr Anne Hart, Dr Suzy Kim, Dr Howard Knuttgen, and Dr Ian Brittain.

References

Blauwet C, Benjamin-Laing H, Stomphorst J, *et al.* (2013) Testing for boosting at the Paralympic Games: policies, results, and future directions. *Br J Sports Med,* 47, 832–837.

Burnham R., Wheeler G., Bhambani Y, *et al.* (1994) Intentional injuction of autonomic dysreflexia among quadriplegic athletes for performance enhancement: efficacy, safety and mechanisms of action. *Clin J Sports Med,* 4, 1–10.

Dauty M, Perrouin VB, Maugars Y, Dubois C, and Mathe JF. (2000) Supralesional and sublesional bone mineral density in spinal cord-injuried patients. *Bone,* 27, 305–309.

International Paralympic Committee Position Statement on Autonomic Dysreflexia and Boosting: London. (2012) *Paralympic Games Operational Management (2013).* International Paralympic Committee.

Krassioukov A. (2012) Autonomic dysreflexia: current evidence related to unstable arterial blood pressure control among athletes with spinal cord injury. *Clin J Sport Med,* 22, 39–45.

Linsenmeyer T, Stone J, and Steins S. (2010) Neurogenic bladder and bowel. In WFrontera and JDe Lisa (eds), *Physical Medicine and Rehabilitation: Principles and Practice* (5th edn, pp. 1369–1370). Lippincott Williams & Wilkins, Philadelphia, PA.

Schwellnus M, Derman W, Jordaan E, *et al.* (2013) Factors associated with illness in athletes participating in the London 2012 Paralympic Games: a prospective cohort study involving 49 910 athlete-days. *Br J Sports Med*, 47, 433–440.

Slade JM, Bickel CS, Modlesky CM, Majumdar S, and Dudley GA. (2005) Trabecular bone is more deteriorated in spinal cord injured vs estrogen-free postmenopausal women. *Osteoporos Int*, 16, 263–272.

United Nations Convention on the Rights of Persons with Disabilities. (2006) *United Nations Enable.* http://www.un.org/disabilities/convention/conventionfull.shtml (accessed on September 24, 2013).

Vestergaard P, Krogh K, Rejnmark L, and Mosekilde L. (1998) Fracture rates and risk factors for fractures in patients with spinal cord injury. *Spinal Cord*, 36, 790.

Webborn N, Willick SE, and Emery CA. (2012) The injury experience at the 2010 Winter Paralympic Games. *Clin J Sport Med*, 22, 3–9.

Willick SE, Webborn N, Emery CA, *et al.* (2013) The epidemiology of injuries at the London 2012 Paralympic Games. *Br J Sports Med*, 47, 426–432.

Recommended reading

Acute Management of Autonomic Dysreflexia. (2001) *Consortium for Spinal Cord Medicine Clinical Practice Guidelines.* Paralyzed Veterans of America.

Battaglino R, Lazzari A, Garshick E, and Morse LR. (2012) Spinal cord injury-induced osteoporosis: pathogenesis and emerging therapies. *Curr Osteoporos Rep*, 10, 278–285.

Bladder Management for Adults with Spinal Cord Injury: A Clinical Practice Guideline for Healthcare Providers. (2006) *Consortium for Spinal Cord Medicine Clinical Practice Guidelines.* Paralyzed Veterans of America.

Blauwet C and Willick SE. (2012) The Paralympic Movement: using sport to promote health, disability rights, and social integration for athletes with disabilities. *PM R*, 4, 851–856.

Brittain I. (2012) *From Stoke Mandeville to Stratford: A History of the Summer Paralympic Games.* Common Ground Publishing, Champaign.

Neurogenic Bowel Management for Adults with Spinal Cord Injury. (1998) *Consortium for Spinal Cord Medicine Clinical Practice Guidelines.* Paralyzed Veterans of America.

Willick SE and Webborn N. (2011) Medicine. In Y Vanlandewijck and W Thompson (eds), *The Paralympic Athlete* (pp. 74–88). Wiley-Blackwell, Sussex.

Index

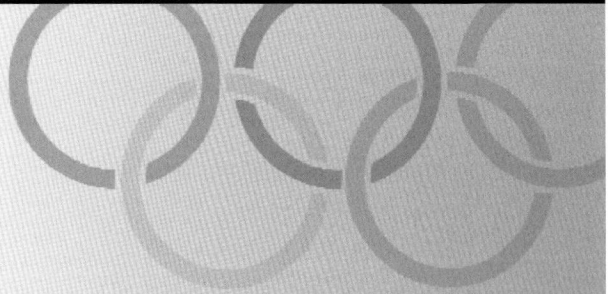

Note: Page numbers with italicised *f*'s and *t*'s refer to figures and tables, respectively.

The Female Athlete, First Edition. Edited by Margo L. Mountjoy. © 2015 International Olympic Committee.
Published 2015 by John Wiley & Sons, Inc.